SYMPTOM GUIDE

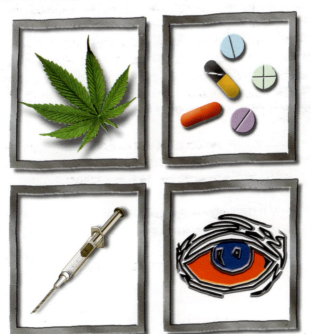

3rd Edition

LawTech
QWIK-CODE

Author: **Ken Whitley**
About the Author: Ken Whitley is a Sergeant with an Orange County Police Agency in CA. Sgt. Whitley is a 29 year police veteran. He is a certified Drug Recognition Expert and a DRE instructor.

Copyright © 1992-2000 *LawTech Publishing Co., Ltd.*
[All rights reserved. No part of this publication may be reproduced, stored in a retrieval system or transmitted, in any form or by any means, electronic, mechanical, photocopying, recording or otherwise without prior written permission from LawTech Publishing Co., Ltd.]

QWIK-CODE is a trademark of *LawTech Publishing Co., Ltd.*

Cover Design: Bridgette Kirkpatrick
Interior Graphic Design: Stuart Ramsey

Published by:
LawTech Publishing Co., Ltd.
1060 Calle Cordillera, Ste. 105
San Clemente, CA 92673
1(949) 498-4815
FAX: 1(949) 498-4858
Web site: *www.lawtech.cc*

SPECIAL THANKS TO THE FOLLOWING PEOPLE FOR THEIR VALUABLE CONTRIBUTIONS TO THIS GUIDE:

Bradley Girard Graphic Design, San Clemente, CA *www.bradleygirard.com*

Jim Mock: *www.drugid.org*

Jim Aumond: Training Director - California Narcotic Officers' Association (CNOA)
www.cnoa.org

Trinka Porrata: Narcotics Detective (Ret.), Drug Consultant.
equus555@worldnet.att.net, or (626)577-5204

Printed in China

p. 256

ISBN: 1-930466-11-0

Table of Contents

Table of Contents i

Qwik Reference Photos 1

Drug I.D. 15

Cannabis
Hashish (Domestic) 16
Hashish (Middle Eastern) 18
HashOil (Domestic) 20
HashOil (Middle Eastern) 22
Marijuana 24
Marijuana Cigarette 26
Marijuana Plant 28
Thai Stick 30

Depressants
Barbiturates 32
Non-Barbiturates 33
Anti-Anxiety Tranquilizers 34
Anti Depressants 35
Anti-Psychotic Tranquilizers 36
Combinations 37
GHB/GHL/GBL 38
Rohypnol 40
Symptoms 42

Hallucinogens
D.M.T. (Dimethyltryptamine) 44
Jimson Weed 46
L.S.D. Lysergic Acid Diethylamide 48
Peyote 50
Psilocybin 52

Table of Contents

Inhalants
Amyl/Butyl Nitrite..**54**
Chlorohydrocarbons **56**
Correction Fluid **58**
Hydrocarbons **60**
Nitrous Oxide..**62**
Additional Inhalants **66**

Narcotics
Codiene **68**
Demerol **70**
Dilaudid **72**
Heroin (Asian-China White) **74**
Heroin (Black Tar) **76**
Heroin (Columbian) **78**
Heroin Paraphernalia **80**
Heroin (Mexican Brown).......................................**82**
Heroin in a balloon **84**
Meperidine **86**
Methadone **88**
Methadone (Dolophine Sulfate) **90**
Methadone Identification Card **92**
Morphine **94**
Opium **96**
Perocet...**98**
Percodan **100**
Additional Narcotics **102**

Phencyclidine
P.C.P. **104**
P.C.P. Liquid..**106**

Table of Contents

Psychedelic Amphetamine
- Ecstasy (XTC) 108
- Ecstasy (XTC) 110

Stimulants
- Amphetamines 112
- Biphetamines 114
- Cocaine (Crack/Freebase) 116
- Cocaine (Crack/Freebase Paraphernalia) 118
- Cocaine (Powder) 120
- Cocaine (Powder Paraphernalia) 122
- Methamphetamine (ICE) 124
- Methamphetamine (Crank or Speed) 126
- Methcathinone 128
- Additional Stimulants 130

Paraphernalia I.D. & Descriptions
- Assorted Smoking Paraphernalia 132
- Bindle 133
- Cocaine Sifter 134
- Copper Scouring Pads 135
- Drug Lab 136
- Freebase Smoking Pipe 137
- Heroin (used cottons, cooker & syringe) 139
- Heroin (Contained in a toy balloon) 140
- Marijuana Roach Clips 141
- Methamphetamine Smoking Pipe (ICE) 142
- Scales 148
- Snorting Spoon 150
- Snorting Tubes 151
- Snorting Vial 152
- Stash Cans 157
- Washback Method 161

Table of Contents

Needle Marks
- Steril Injections **164**
- Unsteril Injections **165**

Weights & Measures
- Equivalant Weights & Measures **168**

Drug Testing
- Drug Testing **170**
- Horizontal Nystagmus Test **171**
- Vertical Nystagmus Test **172**
- Non-Convergence Test **173**
- Standard Field Sobriety Tests **174**
- Field Sobriety Tests **175**
- Walk And Turn **176**
- One Leg Stand **177**
- Finger To the Nose **178**
- Body Fluids Required For Testing **179**
- Length of Time Can Be Detected in Urine **180**

Definitions **182**

Street Slang Glossary **186**

Drug Abuse In The Workplace **228**

Early Warning Signs of Drug Abuse **232**

Gateway Drugs **233**

Drug Statistics **234**

Aircraft Narcotic Smuggling **236**

Resources for Drug Prevention **238**

Index **240**

QWIK REFERENCE I.D. PHOTOS

QWIK REFERENCE I.D. PHOTOS

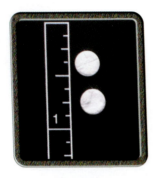

AMPHETAMINES
(pg. 112)

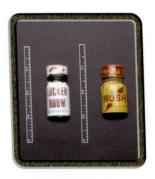

AMYL/BUTYL NITRITE
(pg. 54)

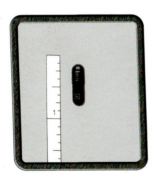

BIPHETAMINES
(pg. 114)

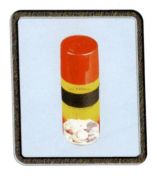

CHLOROHYDROCARBONS
(pg. 56)

QWIK REFERENCE I.D. PHOTOS

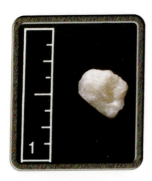

COCAINE (Freebase)
(pg. 156)

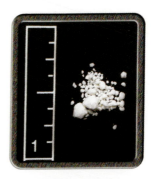

COCAINE (Powder)
(pg. 120)

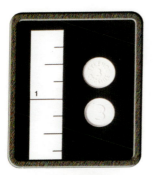

CODEINE (BRAND)
(TYLENOL W/ CODEINE #3)
(pg. 68)

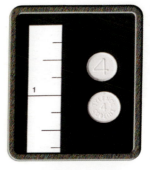

CODEINE (BRAND)
(TYLENOL W/ CODEINE #4)
(pg. 68)

QWIK REFERENCE I.D. PHOTOS

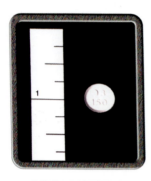

CODEINE (GENERIC)
(TYLENOL W/ CODEINE #3)
(pg. 68)

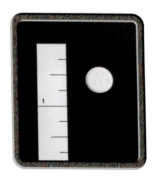

CODEINE (GENERIC)
(TYLENOL W/ CODEINE #4)
(pg. 68)

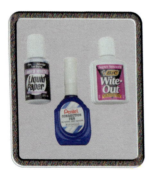

CORRECTION FLUID
(pg. 58)

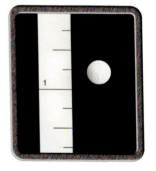

DEMEROL
(pg. 70)

QWIK REFERENCE I.D. PHOTOS

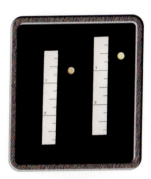

DILAUDID
(pg. 72)

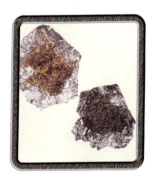

D.M.T.
(Dimethyltryptamine)
(pg. 44)

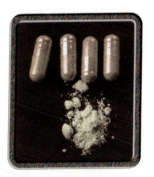

ECSTASY (XTC)
(pg. 108)

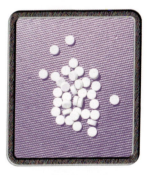

ECSTASY (XTC)
(pg. 110)

QWIK REFERENCE I.D. PHOTOS

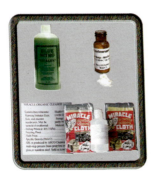

GHB/GHL/GBL
(pg. 38)

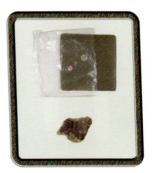

HASHISH
(Domestic)
(pg. 16)

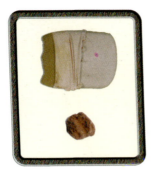

HASHISH
(Middle Eastern)
(pg. 18)

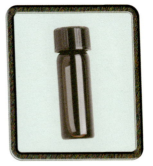

HASHISH OIL
(Domestic)
(pg. 20)

QWIK REFERENCE I.D. PHOTOS

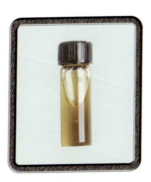

HASHISH OIL
(Middle Eastern)
(pg. 22)

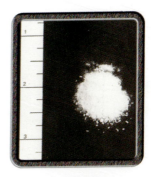

HEROIN
(Asian-China White)
(pg. 74)

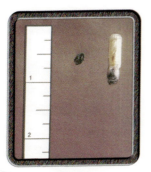

HEROIN
(Black Tar)
(pg. 76)

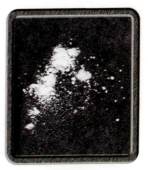

HEROIN
(Columbian)
(pg. 78)

QWIK REFERENCE I.D. PHOTOS

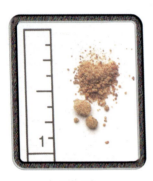

HEROIN
(Mexican Brown)
(pg. 82)

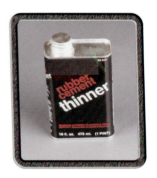

HYDROCARBONS
(pg. 60)

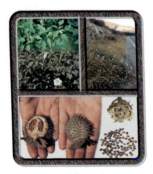

JIMSON WEED
(pg. 46)

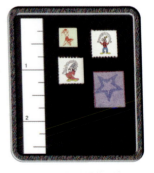

L.S.D. (Lysergic Acid
Diethylamide)
(pg. 48)

QWIK REFERENCE I.D. PHOTOS

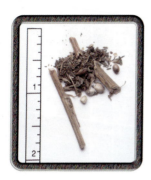

MARIJUANA
(pg. 24)

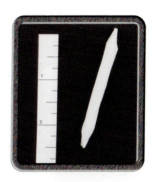

MARIJUANA CIGARETTE
(pg. 26)

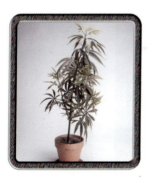

MARIJUANA PLANT
(pg. 28)

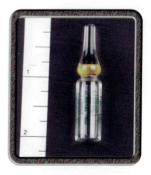

MEPERIDINE
(pg. 86)

QWIK REFERENCE I.D. PHOTOS

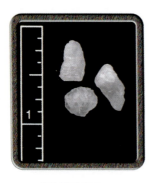

**METHAMPHETAMINE
(ICE)
(pg. 124)**

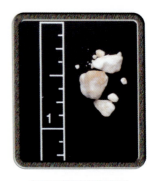

**METHAMPHETAMINE
(Speed or Crank)
(pg. 126)**

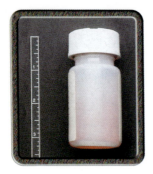

**METHADONE
(pg. 88)**

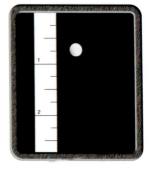

**METHADONE
(Dolophine Sulfate)
(pg. 90)**

QWIK REFERENCE I.D. PHOTOS

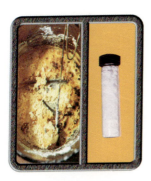

METHCATHINONE
(pg. 128)

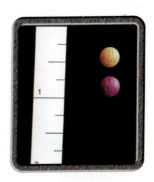

MORPHINE
(pg. 94)

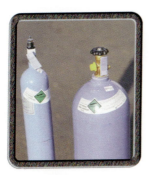

NITROUS OXIDE
(Laughing Gas)
(pg. 62)

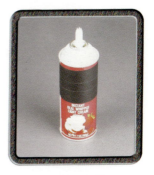

NITROUS OXIDE
(Whipped Cream)
(pg. 64)

CANNABIS

THAI STICK

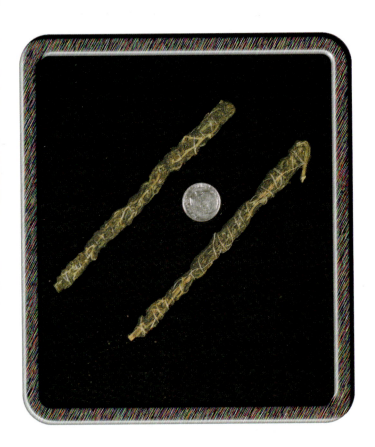

QWIK REFERENCE I.D. PHOTOS

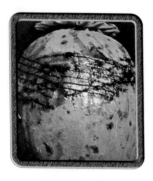

OPIUM (Poppy)
(pg. 96)

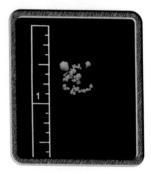

P.C.P.
(Phencyclidine)
(pg. 104)

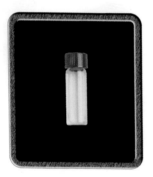

P.C.P. OIL
(Phencyclidine)
(pg. 106)

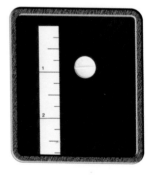

PERCOCET
(pg. 98)

QWIK REFERENCE I.D. PHOTOS

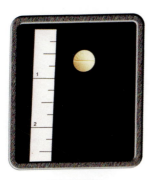
PERCODAN
(pg. 100)

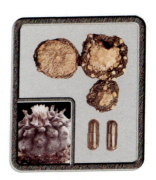
PEYOTE
(pg. 50)

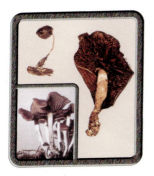
PSILOCYBIN
(Magic Mushrooms)
(pg. 52)

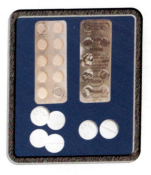
ROHYPNOL
(pg. 40)

QWIK REFERENCE I.D. PHOTOS

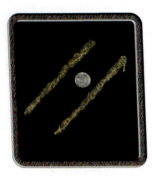

THAI STICK
(pg. 30)

DRUG IDENTIFICATION

CANNABIS

HASHISH
(DOMESTIC)

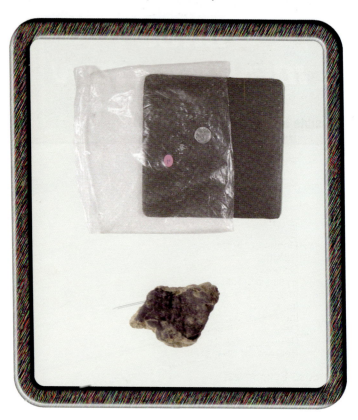

CANNABIS

HASHISH
(DOMESTIC)

Visual Description:
   Solid dark green or gold substance.

Methods of Use:
   Ingested, Smoked

Duration of Effects:
   Onset: 8-10 Seconds   Loaded: 4-6 Hours
   Peak: 10-30 Minutes   Normal: Variable

Possible Effects:
   Nystagmus - No
   Pupils - Normal (Possibly Dilated)
   Pulse - Elevated
   Blood Pressure - Elevated
   Body Temperature - Near Normal
   Non-Convergence - Yes

   Bloodshot Eyes
   Body Tremors
   Debris in Mouth
   Difficulty Concentrating
   Disoriented
   Eyelid Tremors
   Impaired Divided Attention
   Impaired Time/Distance Perception
   Increased Appetite
   Odor of Burning Marijuana
   Rebound Dilation
   Relaxed Inhibitions

Overdose Symptoms:
   Fatigue
   Paranoia
   Psychosis

Body Fluids Required For Testing: Blood

HASHISH
(MIDDLE EASTERN)

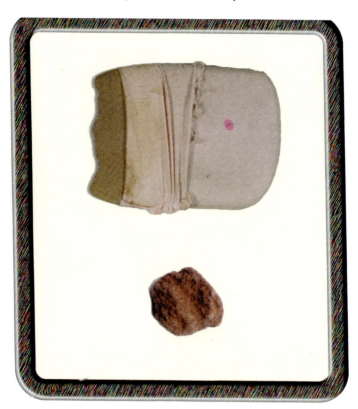

CANNABIS

HASHISH
(MIDDLE EASTERN)

Visual Description:
Solid dark green or gold substance.

Methods of Use:
Ingested, Smoked

Duration of Effects:
Onset: 8-10 Seconds   Loaded: 4-6 Hours
Peak: 10-30 Minutes   Normal: Variable

Possible Effects:
Nystagmus - No
Pupils - Normal (Possibly Dilated)
Pulse - Elevated
Blood Pressure - Elevated
Body Temperature - Near Normal
Non-Convergence - Yes

Bloodshot Eyes
Body Tremors
Debris in Mouth
Difficulty Concentrating
Disoriented
Eyelid Tremors
Impaired Divided Attention
Impaired Time/Distance Perception
Increased Appetite
Odor of Burning Marijuana
Rebound Dilation
Relaxed Inhibitions

Overdose Symptoms:
Fatigue
Paranoia
Psychosis

Body Fluids Required For Testing: Blood

CANNABIS

HASHISH OIL
(DOMESTIC)

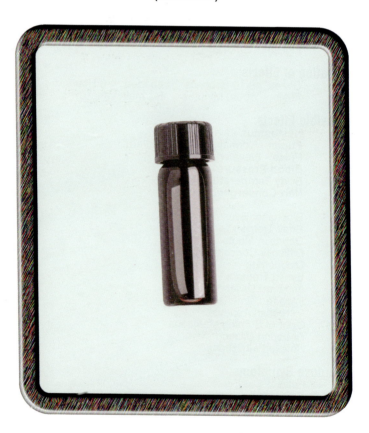

CANNABIS

HASHISH OIL
(DOMESTIC)

Visual Description:
Concentrated, thick liquid dark in color.

Methods of Use:
Smoked - Mixed with tobacco or marijuana.

Duration of Effects:
Onset: 8-10 Seconds   Loaded: 4-6 Hours
Peak: 10-30 Minutes   Normal: Variable

Possible Effects:
Nystagmus - No
Pupils - Normal (Possibly Dilated)
Pulse - Elevated
Blood Pressure - Elevated
Body Temperature - Near Normal
Non-Convergence - Yes

Bloodshot Eyes
Body Tremors
Debris in Mouth
Difficulty Concentrating
Disoriented
Eyelid Tremors
Impaired Divided Attention
Impaired Time/Distance Perception
Increased Appetite
Odor of Burning Marijuana
Rebound Dilation
Relaxed Inhibitions

Overdose Symptoms:
Fatigue
Paranoia
Psychosis

Body Fluids Required For Testing: Blood

CANNABIS

HASHISH OIL
(MIDDLE EASTERN)

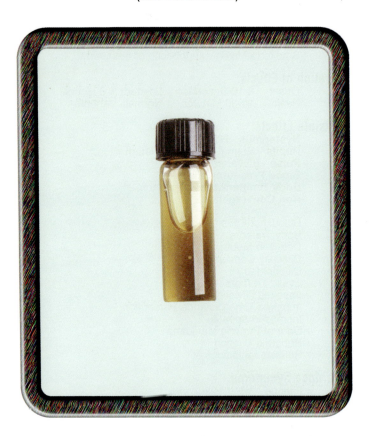

HASHISH OIL
(MIDDLE EASTERN)

Visual Description:
> Concentrated, thick liquid gold in color.

Methods of Use:
> Smoked - Mixed with tobacco or marijuana.

Duration of Effects:
> Onset: 8-10 Seconds   Loaded: 4-6 Hours
> Peak: 10-30 Minutes   Normal: Variable

Possible Effects:
> **Nystagmus -** No
> **Pupils -** Normal (Possibly Dilated)
> **Pulse -** Elevated
> **Blood Pressure -** Elevated
> **Body Temperature -** Near Normal
> **Non-Convergence -** Yes
>
> Bloodshot Eyes
> Body Tremors
> Debris in Mouth
> Difficulty Concentrating
> Disoriented
> Eyelid Tremors
> Impaired Divided Attention
> Impaired Time/Distance Perception
> Increased Appetite
> Odor of Burning Marijuana
> Rebound Dilation
> Relaxed Inhibitions

Overdose Symptoms:
> Fatigue
> Paranoia
> Psychosis

Body Fluids Required For Testing: Blood

CANNABIS

MARIJUANA

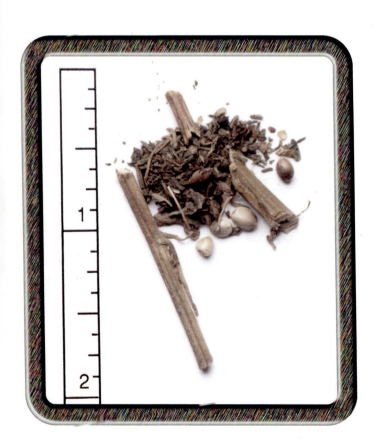

CANNABIS

MARIJUANA

Visual Description:
A dried, green leafy substance mixed with stems and possibly seeds.

Methods of Use:
Ingested, Smoked

Duration of Effects:
Onset: 8-10 Seconds Loaded: 2-3 Hours
Peak: 10-30 Minutes Normal: Variable

Possible Effects:
Nystagmus - No
Pupils - Normal (Possibly Dilated)
Pulse - Elevated
Blood Pressure - Elevated
Body Temperature - Near Normal
Non-Convergence - Yes

Bloodshot Eyes
Body Tremors
Debris in Mouth
Difficulty Concentrating
Disoriented
Eyelid Tremors
Impaired Divided Attention
Impaired Time/Distance Perception
Increased Appetite
Odor of Burning Marijuana
Rebound Dilation
Relaxed Inhibitions

Overdose Symptoms:
Fatigue
Paranoia
Psychosis

Body Fluids Required For Testing: Blood

CANNABIS

MARIJUANA CIGARETTE

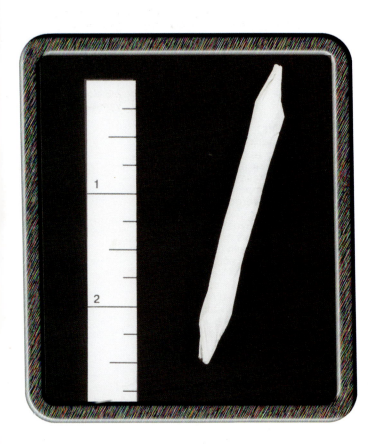

CANNABIS

MARIJUANA CIGARETTE

Visual Description:
A dried, green leafy substance mixed with stems and possibly seeds hand-rolled into a cigarette (joint).

Methods of Use:
Smoked

Duration of Effects:
Onset: 8-10 Seconds Loaded: 2-3 Hours
Peak: 10-30 Minutes Normal: Variable

Possible Effects:
Nystagmus - No
Pupils - Normal (Possibly Dilated)
Pulse - Elevated
Blood Pressure - Elevated
Body Temperature - Near Normal
Non-Convergence - Yes

Bloodshot Eyes
Body Tremors
Debris in Mouth
Difficulty Concentrating
Disoriented
Eyelid Tremors
Impaired Divided Attention
Impaired Time/Distance Perception
Increased Appetite
Odor of Burning Marijuana
Rebound Dilation
Relaxed Inhibitions

Overdose Symptoms:
Fatigue
Paranoia
Psychosis

Body Fluids Required For Testing: Blood

CANNABIS

MARIJUANA PLANT

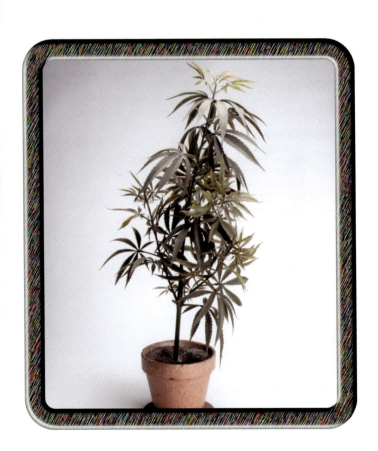

CANNABIS

MARIJUANA PLANT

Visual Description:
Stalked green plant with saw-like or serrated edged leaves. Usually an odd number of leaves.

Methods of Use:
Ingested, Smoked

Duration of Effects:
Onset: 8-10 Seconds   Loaded: 2-3 Hours
Peak: 10-30 Minutes   Normal: Variable

Possible Effects:
Nystagmus - No
Pupils - Normal (Possibly Dilated)
Pulse - Elevated
Blood Pressure - Elevated
Body Temperature - Near Normal
Non-Convergence - Yes

Bloodshot Eyes
Body Tremors
Debris in Mouth
Difficulty Concentrating
Disoriented
Eyelid Tremors
Impaired Divided Attention
Impaired Time/Distance Perception
Increased Appetite
Odor of Burning Marijuana
Rebound Dilation
Relaxed Inhibitions

Overdose Symptoms:
Fatigue
Paranoia
Psychosis

Body Fluids Required For Testing: Blood

CANNABIS

THAI STICK

Visual Description:
High grade marijuana tied to thin sticks with string or fishing line.

Methods of Use:
Ingested, Smoked

Duration of Effects:
Onset: 8-10 Seconds   Loaded: 4-6 Hours
Peak: 10-30 Minutes   Normal: Variable

Possible Effects:
Nystagmus - No
Pupils - Normal (Possibly Dilated)
Pulse - Elevated
Blood Pressure - Elevated
Body Temperature - Near Normal
Non-Convergence - Yes

Bloodshot Eyes
Body Tremors
Debris in Mouth
Difficulty Concentrating
Disoriented
Eyelid Tremors
Euphoria
Impaired Divided Attention
Impaired Time/Distance Perception
Increased Appetite
Odor of Burning Marijuana
Rebound Dilation
Relaxed Inhibitions

Overdose Symptoms:
Fatigue
Paranoia
Psychosis

Body Fluids Required For Testing: Blood

DEPRESSANTS

BARBITURATES

Amobarbital
Amosecobarbital
Mephobarbital
Pentobarbital
Phenobarbital
Secobarbital
Sodium Butabarbital
Talbutal

Visual Description:
    Red, Yellow & Blue Capsules
    Red & Blue Capsules

Methods of Use:
    Ingested, Injected, Snorted

Trade Names:

Amytal	Mebaral
Buticaps	Nembutal
Butisol	Seconal
Lotusate	Tuinal

Body Fluids Required For Testing: Blood (10ML 2 Vacutainer Tubes)

DEPRESSANTS

NON-BARBITURATES

Chloral Hydrate
Ethchlorvynol
Ethinamate
Glutethimide
Meprobamate
Methaqualone
Methyprylon
Paraldehyde

Visual Description:
Tablets

Methods of Use:
Ingested, Injected, Snorted

Trade Names:
Doriden	Placidyl
Equanil	Quaalude
Miltown	Valmid
Noctec	

Body Fluids Required For Testing: Blood (10ML-2 Vacutainer Tubes)

DEPRESSANTS

ANTI-ANXIETY TRANQUILIZERS

Alprazolam
Chlordiazepoxide
Clorazepate
Diazepam
Diphenhydramine Hydrochloride
Flurazepam
Hydroxyzine
Lorazepam
Oxazepam
Phenytoin Sodium
Prazepam

Visual Description:
Tablets

Methods of Use:
Ingested, Injected, Snorted

Trade Names:

Atarax	Librium	Valium
Ativan	Reposans-10	Vazepam
Centrax	Serax	Vistaril
Dalmane	Tranxene	Xanax

Body Fluids Required For Testing: Blood (10ML-2 Vacutainer Tubes)

DEPRESSANTS

ANTI-DEPRESSANTS

Amitriptyline Hydrochloride
Desipramine
Doxepin Hydrochloride
Imipramine
Isocarboxazid
Nortriptyline
Phenelzine
Tranylcypromine
Trazodone

Visual Description:
  Tablets

Methods of Use:
  Ingested, Injected, Snorted

Trade Names:
  Adapin   Nardil
  Desyrel   Norpramine
  Elavil   Pamelor
  Marplan   Parnate
              Tofranil

Body Fluids Required For Testing: Blood (10Ml-2 Vacutainer Tubes)

DEPRESSANTS

ANTI-PSYCHOTIC TRANQUILIZERS

Chlorpromazine
Droperidol
Fluphenazine Hydrochloride
Haloperidol
Lithium Carbonate
Lithium Citrate
Perphenazine
Promazine
Thioridazine

Visual Description:
  Tablets

Methods of Use:
  Ingested, Injected, Snorted

Trade Names:
  Cibalith
  Eskalith
  Haldol
  Inapsine
  Mellaril
  Permitil
  Proxlixin
  Sparine
  Thorazine
  Trilafon

Body Fluids Required For Testing: Blood (10ML-2 Vacutainer Tubes)

DEPRESSANTS

COMBINATIONS

Chlordiazepoxide & Amitriptyline
Chlordiazepoxide Hydrochloride & Clidinium Bromide
Perphenazine & Amitriptyline Hydrochloride

Visual Description:
   Tablets

Methods of Use:
   Ingested, Injected, Snorted

Trade Names:
   Librax
   Limbitrol
   Triavil

Body Fluids Required For Testing: Blood

DEPRESSANTS

GHB/GHL/GBL

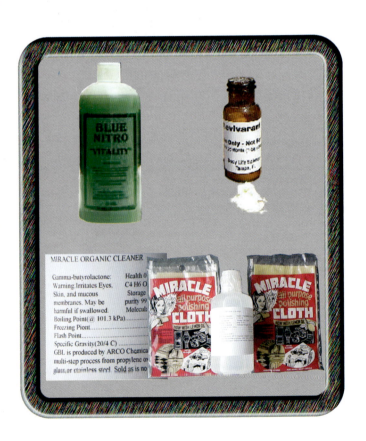

DEPRESSANTS

GHB/GHL/GBL

Visual Description: GBL can be produced in the form of a liquid with a clear or yellowish gold color and a salty taste. It also is produced in a tablet or capsule form or a white powder.

Duration of Effects:
Onset: 10-15 minutes
Duration: 3-5 hours

Method of Use:
Often used in combination with alcohol

Possible Effects:
Nystagmus - Yes (High Levels/Possible Vertical Nystagmus)
Pupils - Near Normal
Pulse - Below Normal
Blood Pressure - Below Normal
Body Temperature - Near Normal
Non-Convergence - Yes

Disoriented
Droopy Eye Lids (Ptosis)
Drowsiness
Drunken Behavior (Without Odor of Alcohol)
Gait Ataxia
Pupils Slow to React
Slurred Speech

Overdose Symptoms:
Amnesia
Cold & Clammy Skin
Coma
Loss of Bowel Control
Nausea
Shallow Respiration
Vomiting
Weak & Rapid Pulse
Death

Body Fluids Required For Testing:
Blood (3-5 hrs.) Urine (12 hrs.)

DEPRESSANTS

ROHYPNOL

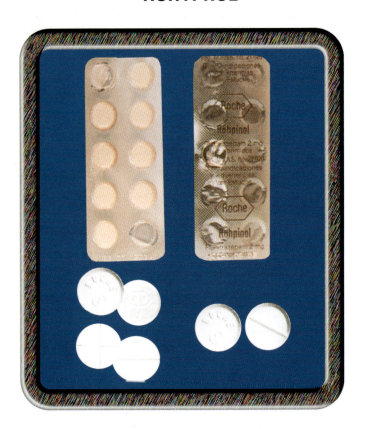

DEPRESSANTS

ROHYPNOL

Visual Description: Single or double scored white tablet with mfr. name as either ROCHE or ⟨ RH ⟩ and with the number 1 (1 = 1mg) or 2 (2 = 2mg)

Method of Use: Usually mixed in a drink

Duration of Effects:
  Onset   10-15 minutes
  Loaded   6-10 hours

Possible Effects:
Nystagmus - Yes (High Levels/Possible Vertical Nystagmus)
Pupils - Near Normal
Pulse - Below Normal
Blood Pressure - Below Normal
Body Temperature - Near Normal
Non-Convergence - Yes

Amnesia
Bloodshot, watery eyes
Confusion
Disinhibition
Dizziness
Droopy Eye Lids (Ptosis)
Drunken Behavior
Slurred Speech
Excitability/Aggression

Overdose Symptoms:
Drowsiness
Mental Confusion
Lethargy
Poor Coordination
Reduced Reflexes

NOTE: Because Rohypnol produces amnesia in the non-frequent user, and is oderless, colorless, tasteless and dissolves very quickly, it has become infamous as the "date rape" drug. The manufacturer, Hoffman-La Roche, is seeking approval to add a color releasing agent to the pill, turning beer green and other drinks blue. Though typically white in color Rohypnol pills recently seized in Egypt were of a brownish-pink tint, indicating a counterfeit product.

Body Fluids Required For Testing: Blood

DEPRESSANTS

SYMPTOMS

Duration of Effects:
- Barbiturates: 1-16 Hours
- Quaaludes: 4-8 Hours
- Tranquilizers: 4-8 Hours

Possible Effects:
- **Nystagmus** - Yes (High Levels/Possible Vertical Nystagmus)
- **Pupils** - Near Normal
- **Pulse** - Below Normal
- **Blood Pressure** - Below Normal
- **Body Temperature** - Near Normal
- **Non-Convergence** - Yes

- Disoriented
- Droopy Eye Lids (Ptosis)
- Drowsiness
- Drunken Behavior (Without Odor of Alcohol)
- Gait Ataxia
- Pupils Slow to React
- Slurred Speech

NOTE: Methaqualone Pupils - Dilated
                       Pulse - Elevated

Alcohol Pulse - Elevated
         Blood Pressure - Elevated

Overdose Symptoms:
- Cold & Clammy Skin
- Coma
- Shallow Respiration
- Weak & Rapid Pulse
- Death

Body Fluids Required For Testing: Blood

DEPRESSANTS

HALLUCINOGENS

D.M.T.
(DIMETHYLTRYPTAMINE)

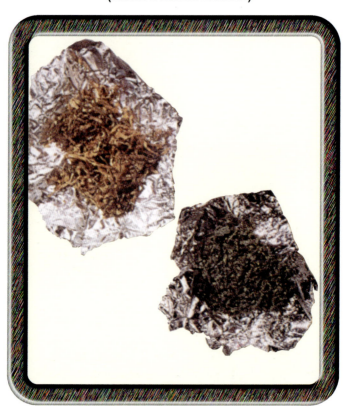

HALLUCINOGENS

D.M.T.
(DIMETHYLTRYPTAMINE)

Visual Description:
Capsule, Liquid, Pill, Tablet

Methods of Use:
Ingested, Injected, Smoked, Snorted

Duration of Effects:
Loaded: 1 Hour

Possible Effects:
Nystagmus - No
Pupils - Dilated
Pulse - Elevated
Blood Pressure - Elevated
Body Temperature - Elevated
Non-Convergence - No

Blank Stare
Body Tremors
Dazed
Disoriented
Flashbacks
Hallucinations
Impaired Divided Attention
Mood Changes
Memory Loss
Muscle Tension
Nausea
Perspiring
Sleeplessness
Synesthesia

Overdose Symptoms:
Bizarre Behavior
Long, Intense Trips
Psychosis
Violence
Death

Note: Sometimes referred to as a "Business Man's Lunch".

Body Fluids Required For Testing: Urine

NOTE: If you are unsure, it is advisable to take blood as the user may be under the influence of a combination of drugs.

HALLUCINOGENS

JIMSON WEED

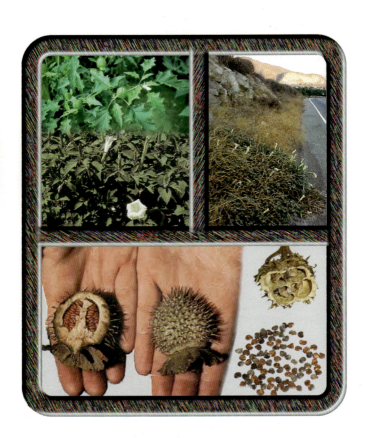

HALLUCINOGENS

JIMSON WEED

Visual Description:
Flower pods containing seeds which are consumed. The plant grows wild in Southern California. Jimson is a green bush with white trumpet shaped flowers. The pods when dried, are a light green in color and prickely.

Methods of Use:
Ingested

Duration of Effects:
Variable

Possible Effects:
Nystagmus - No
Pupils - Dilated
Pulse - Elevated
Blood Pressure - Elevated
Body Temperature - Elevated
Non-Convergence - No

- Blank Stare
- Body Tremors
- Dazed
- Disoriented
- Flashbacks
- Hallucinations
- Impaired Divided Attention
- Mood Changes
- Memory Loss
- Muscle Tension
- Nausea
- Perspiring
- Sleeplessness
- Synesthesia

Overdose Symptoms:
- Bizarre Behavior
- Psychosis
- Violence
- Death

Body Fluids Required For Testing: No Test

HALLUCINOGENS

L.S.D.
(LYSERGIC ACID DIETHYLAMIDE)

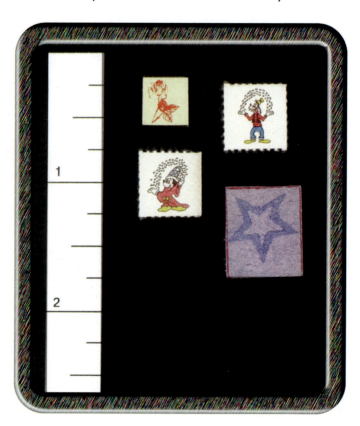

HALLUCINOGENS

L.S.D.
(LYSERGIC ACID DIETHYLAMIDE)

Visual Description:
Square, perforated, impregnated blotter paper, often with cartoon characters on them.

Methods of Use:
Ingested

Duration of Effects:
Variable

Possible Effects:
Nystagmus - No
Pupils - Dilated
Pulse - Elevated
Blood Pressure - Elevated
Body Temperature - Elevated
Non-Convergence - No

Blank Stare
Body Tremors
Dazed
Disoriented
Flashbacks
Hallucinations
Impaired Divided Attention
Mood Changes
Memory Loss
Muscle Tension
Nausea
Perspiring
Sleeplessness
Synesthesia

Overdose Symptoms:
Bizarre Behavior
Long, Intense Trips
Psychosis
Violence
Death

Body Fluids Required For Testing: No Test

HALLUCINOGENS

PEYOTE

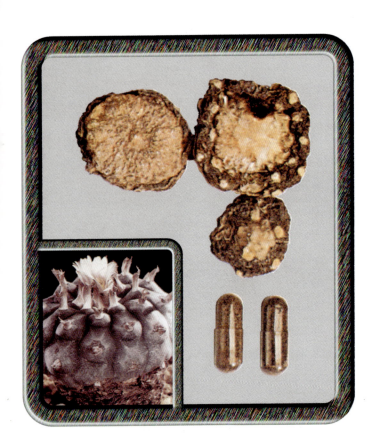

HALLUCINOGENS

PEYOTE

Visual Description:
 Capsules, Hard Brown Discs, Tablets

Methods of Use:
 Capsules & Tablets - Ingested
 Discs - Chewed, smoked & swallowed.
 Ingested in soup or tea form.

Duration of Effects:
 Variable

Possible Effects:
 Nystagmus - No
 Pupils - Dilated
 Pulse - Elevated
 Blood Pressure - Elevated
 Body Temperature - Elevated
 Non-Convergence - No

- Body Tremors
- Dazed
- Disoriented
- Flashbacks
- Hallucinations
- Impaired Divided Attention
- Memory Loss
- Mood Changes
- Muscle Tension
- Nausea
- Rancid Breath
- Sleeplessness
- Synesthesia

Overdose Symptoms:
 Bizarre Behavior
 Long, Intense Trips
 Psychosis
 Violence
 Death

Body Fluids Required For Testing: Blood

HALLUCINOGENS

PSILOCYBIN
(MAGIC MUSHROOMS)

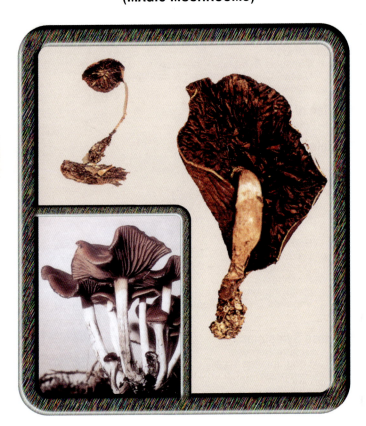

HALLUCINOGENS

PSILOCYBIN
(MAGIC MUSHROOMS)

Visual Description:
Fresh or Dried Mushrooms

Methods of Use:
Chewed and Swallowed

Duration of Effects:
Variable

Possible Effects:
Nystagmus - No
Pupils - Dilated
Pulse - Elevated
Blood Pressure - Elevated
Body Temperature - Elevated
Non-Convergence - No

- Body Tremors
- Dazed
- Disoriented
- Flashbacks
- Hallucinations
- Impaired Divided Attention
- Memory Loss
- Muscle Tension
- Nausea
- Sleeplessness
- Synesthesia

Overdose Symptoms:
- Bizarre Behavior
- Long, Intense Trips
- Psychosis
- Violence
- Death

Body Fluids Required For Testing: Blood

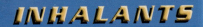

INHALANTS

AMYL/BUTYL NITRITE

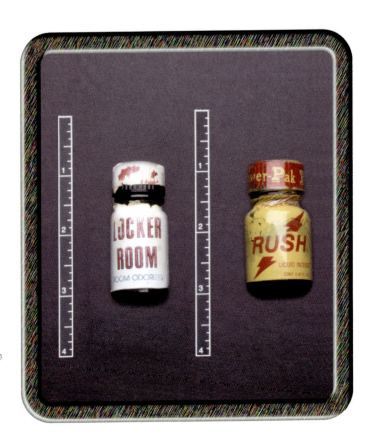

INHALANTS

AMYL/BUTYL NITRITE

Visual Description:
Packaged in small bottles. (Sold under brand names: "Locker Room", "Rush", "Come", etc. Sold as room deodorizers.)

Methods of Use:
Vapors Inhaled

Duration of Effects:
Variable

Possible Effects:
Nystagmus - Depends on Substance
Pupils - Normal or Possibly Dilated
Pulse - Elevated
Blood Pressure - Elevated
Body Temperature - Depends on Substance
Non-Convergence - Possibly

Confusion
Disoriented
Headaches
Odor of Substance
Slurred Speech

Overdose Symptoms:
Coma
Death

Body Fluids Required For Testing: Blood

NOTE: Long term use can cause weight loss, fatigue, and muscle fatigue. Consistent inhaling of vapors can, over time, permanently damage the nervous system.

INHALANTS

CHLOROHYDROCARBONS

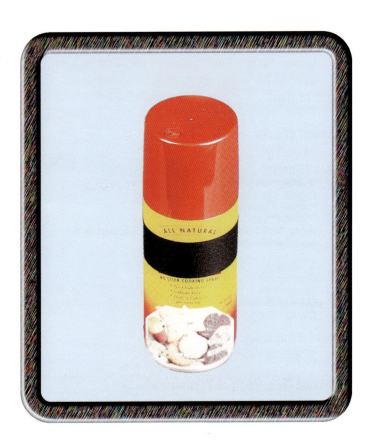

INHALANTS

CHLOROHYDROCARBONS

Visual Description:
　　Aerosol Spray Cans

Methods of Use:
　　Vapors Inhaled

Duration of Effects:
　　Variable

Possible Effects:
　　Nystagmus - Depends on Substance
　　Pupils - Normal or Possibly Dilated
　　Pulse - Elevated
　　Blood Pressure - Elevated
　　Body Temperature - Depends on Substance
　　Non-Convergence - Possibly

　　Confusion
　　Disoriented
　　Impaired Divided Attention
　　Odor of Substance
　　Slurred Speech

Overdose Symptoms:
　　Coma
　　Death

Body Fluids Required For Testing: Blood

NOTE: Long term use can cause weight loss, fatigue, and muscle fatigue. Consistent inhaling of vapors can, over time, permanently damage the nervous system.

INHALANTS

CORRECTION FLUID

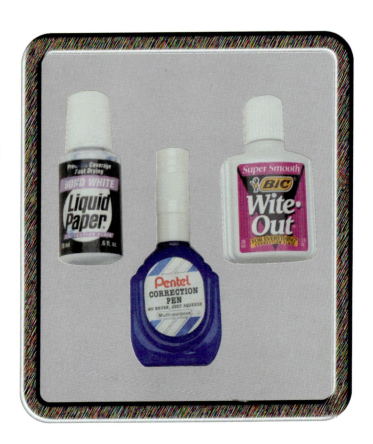

INHALANTS

CORRECTION FLUID

Visual Description:
> White liquid packaged in small bottles.

Methods of Use:
> Vapors Inhaled

Duration of Effects:
> Variable

Possible Effects:
> **Nystagmus -** Depends on Substance
> **Pupils -** Normal or Possibly Dilated
> **Pulse -** Elevated
> **Blood Pressure -** Elevated
> **Body Temperature -** Depends on Substance
> **Non-Convergence -** Possibly
>
> Confusion
> Disoriented
> Impaired Divided Attention
> Odor of Substance
> Slurred Speech

Overdose Symptoms:
> Coma
> Death

Body Fluids Required For Testing: Blood

NOTE: Long term use can cause weight loss, fatigue, and muscle fatigue. Consistent inhaling of vapors can, over time, permanently damage the nervous system.

INHALANTS

HYDROCARBONS

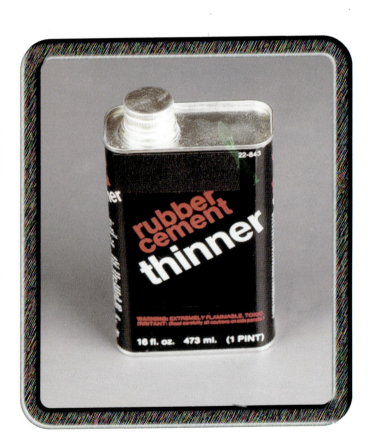

INHALANTS

HYDROCARBONS

Visual Description:
Cans of aerosol propellants, gasoline, glue, paint thinner.

Methods of Use:
Vapors Inhaled

Duration of Effects:
Variable

Possible Effects:
Nystagmus - Depends on Substance
Pupils - Normal or Possibly Dilated
Pulse - Elevated
Blood Pressure - Elevated
Body Temperature - Depends on Substance
Non-Convergence - Possibly

Confusions
Disoriented
Impaired Divided Attention
Odor of Substance
Slurred Speech

Overdose Symptoms:
Coma
Death

Body Fluids Required For Testing: Blood

NOTE: Long term use can cause weight loss, fatigue, and muscle fatigue. Consistent inhaling of vapors can, over time, permanently damage the nervous system.

NITROUS OXIDE
(LAUGHING GAS)

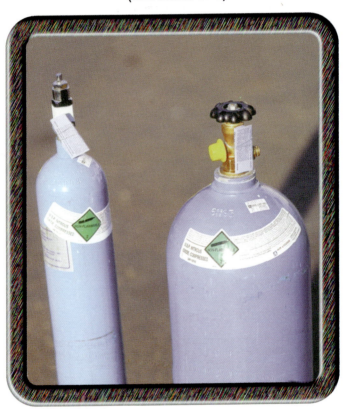

INHALANTS

NITROUS OXIDE
(LAUGHING GAS)

Visual Description:
Small metal cylinder with a balloon or pipe.

Methods of Use:
Vapors Inhaled

Duration of Effects:
Variable

Possible Effects:
Nystagmus - Depends on Substance
Pupils - Normal or Possibly Dilated
Pulse - Elevated
Blood Pressure - Elevated
Body Temperature - Depends on Substance
Non-Convergence - Possibly

Confusion
Disoriented
Impaired Divided Attention
Odor of Substance
Slurred Speech

Overdose Symptoms:
Coma
Death

Body Fluids Required For Testing: Blood

NOTE: Long term use can cause weight loss, fatigue, and muscle fatigue. Consistent inhaling of vapors can, over time, permanently damage the nervous system.

INHALANTS

NITROUS OXIDE
(WHIPPED CREAM)

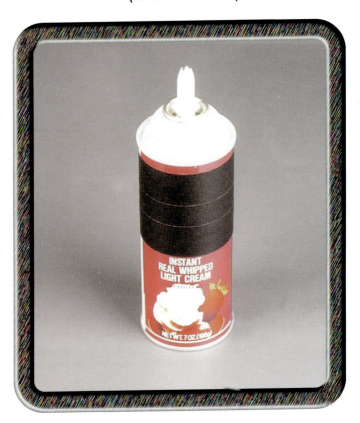

INHALANTS

NITROUS OXIDE
(WHIPPED CREAM)

Visual Description:
Propellant for whipped cream aerosol can.

Methods of Use:
Vapors Inhaled

Duration of Effects:
Variable

Possible Effects:
Nystagmus - Depends on Substance
Pupils - Normal or Possibly Dilated
Pulse - Elevated
Blood Pressure - Elevated
Body Temperature - Depends on Substance
Non-Convergence - Possibly

Confusion
Disoriented
Impaired Divided Attention
Odor of Substance
Slurred Speech

Overdose Symptoms:
Coma
Death

Body Fluids Required For Testing: Blood

NOTE: Long term use can cause weight loss, fatigue, and muscle fatigue. Consistent inhaling of vapors can, over time, permanently damage the nervous system.

INHALANTS

ADDITIONAL INHALANTS

Aerosols
Brush Cleaner
Chloroform
CO_2 Cartridges
Computer Keyboard Dusters
Cooking Spray
Empty Aerosol Cans
Ether
Petroleum Products
Ping Pong Ball Gas
Spray Paints (Silver)

NOTE: Due to the overwhelming amount of various inhalants, it is practically impossible to pinpoint what substance a subject may be under the influence of.

INHALANTS

CODEINE

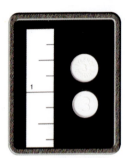

TYLENOL W/ CODEINE #3
(Brand Name)

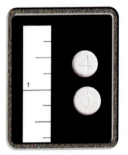

TYLENOL W/ CODEINE #4
(Brand Name)

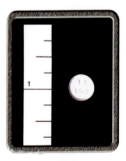

TYLENOL W/ CODEINE #3
(Generic)

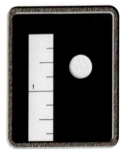

TYLENOL W/ CODEINE #4
(Generic)S

NARCOTICS

CODEINE

Visual Description:
Capsules, Dark Liquid (varying in thickness), Tablets

Methods of Use:
Ingested, Injected, Snorted

Duration of Effects:
Loaded: 4-6 Hours

Possible Effects:
Nystagmus - No
Pupils - Constricted
Pulse - Below Normal
Blood Pressure - Below Normal
Body Temperature - Normal/Below Normal
Non-Convergence - No

Depressed Reflexes
Droopy Eyelids (Ptosis)
Drowsiness
Dry Mouth
Euphoria
Fresh Puncture Marks
Impaired Divided Attention
Low, Raspy Voice
Nausea
Poor Muscle Coordination
Profuse Scratching
Vomiting

Overdose Symptoms:
Cold, Clammy Skin
Convulsions
Rapid, Weak pulse
Slow, Shallow Breathing
Coma
Death

Body Fluids Required For Testing: Urine (20cc) Blood is preferred.

NOTE: If you are unsure, it is advisable to take blood as the user may be under the influence of a combination of drugs.

NOTE: Tolerance to narcotics develops quickly making drug dependence very likely.

NARCOTICS

DEMORAL

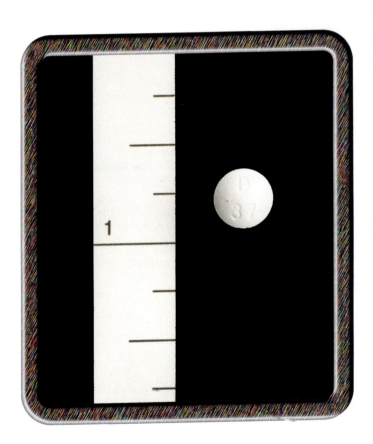

NARCOTICS

DEMEROL

Visual Description:
Tablets, Clear Liquid

Methods of Use:
Ingested, Injected, Snorted

Duration of Effects:
Loaded: 4-6 Hours

Possible Effects:
Nystagmus - No
Pupils - Normal
Pulse - Below Normal
Blood Pressure - Below Normal
Body Temperature - Normal/Below Normal
Non-Convergence - No

Depressed Reflexes
Droopy Eyelids (Ptosis)
Drowsiness
Dry Mouth
Euphoria
Fresh Puncture Marks
Impaired Divided Attention
Low, Raspy Voice
Nausea
Poor Muscle Coordination
Profuse Scratching
Vomiting

Overdose Symptoms:
Cold, Clammy Skin
Convulsions
Rapid, Weak pulse
Slow, Shallow Breathing
Coma
Death

Body Fluids Required For Testing: Urine (20cc) Blood is preferred.

NOTE: If you are unsure, it is advisable to take blood as the user may be under the influence of a combination of drugs.

NOTE: Tolerance to narcotics develops quickly making drug dependence very likely.

DILAUDID

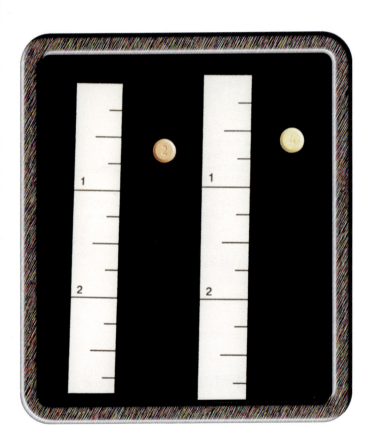

NARCOTICS

DILAUDID

Visual Description:
Tablets, Snorted

Methods of Use:
Ingested

Duration of Effects:
Loaded: 4-6 Hours

Possible Effects:
- **Nystagmus -** No
- **Pupils -** Constricted
- **Pulse -** Below Normal
- **Blood Pressure -** Below Normal
- **Body Temperature -** Normal/Below Normal
- **Non-Convergence -** No

- Depressed Reflexes
- Droopy Eyelids (Ptosis)
- Drowsiness
- Dry Mouth
- Euphoria
- Fresh Puncture Marks
- Impaired Divided Attention
- Low, Raspy Voice
- Nausea
- Poor Muscle Coordination
- Profuse Scratching
- Vomiting

Overdose Symptoms:
- Cold, Clammy Skin
- Convulsions
- Rapid, Weak pulse
- Slow, Shallow Breathing
- Coma
- Death

Body Fluids Required For Testing: Urine (20cc) Blood is preferred.

NOTE: If you are unsure, it is advisable to take blood as the user may be under the influence of a combination of drugs.

NOTE: Tolerance to narcotics develops quickly making drug dependence very likely.

HEROIN
(ASIAN-CHINA WHITE)

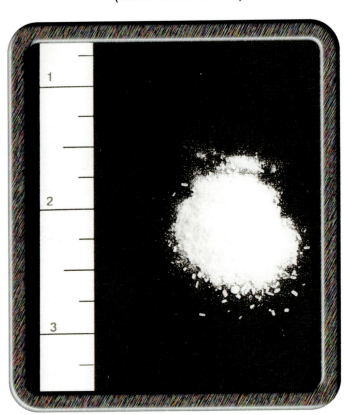

NARCOTICS

HEROIN
(ASIAN-CHINA WHITE)

Visual Description:
White powdered substance.

Methods of Use:
Ingested, Injected, Snorted

Duration of Effects:
Loaded: 4-6 Hours

Possible Effects:
Nystagmus - No
Pupils - Constricted
Pulse - Below Normal
Blood Pressure - Below Normal
Body Temperature - Normal/Below Normal
Non-Convergence - No

- Depressed Reflexes
- Droopy Eyelids (Ptosis)
- Drowsiness
- Dry Mouth
- Euphoria
- Fresh Puncture Marks
- Impaired Divided Attention
- Low, Raspy Voice
- Nausea
- Poor Muscle Coordination
- Profuse Scratching
- Vomiting

Overdose Symptoms:
- Cold, Clammy Skin
- Coma
- Convulsions
- Rapid, Weak pulse
- Slow, Shallow Breathing

Body Fluids Required For Testing: Urine (20cc) Blood is preferred.

NOTE: If you are unsure, it is advisable to take blood as the user may be under the influence of a combination of drugs.

NOTE: Tolerance to narcotics develops quickly making drug dependence very likely.

HEROIN
(BLACK TAR)

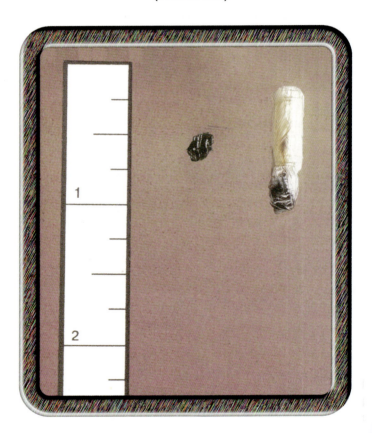

NARCOTICS

HEROIN
(BLACK TAR)

Visual Description:
Black tar-like substance with a vinegar odor.

Methods of Use:
Injected, Ingested, Smoked

Duration of Effects:
Loaded: 4-6 Hours

Possible Effects:
- **Nystagmus -** No
- **Pupils -** Constricted
- **Pulse -** Below Normal
- **Blood Pressure -** Below Normal
- **Body Temperature -** Normal/Below Normal
- **Non-Convergence -** No

Depressed Reflexes
Droopy Eyelids (Ptosis)
Drowsiness
Dry Mouth
Euphoria
Profuse Scratching
Fresh Puncture Marks
Impaired Divided Attention
Low, Raspy Voice
Nausea
Poor Motor Coordination
Vomiting

Overdose Symptoms:
Cold, Clammy Skin
Convulsions
Rapid, Weak Pulse
Slow, Shallow Breathing
Coma
Death

Body Fluids Required For Testing: Urine (20cc) Blood is preferred.

NOTE: If you are unsure, it is advisable to take blood as the user may be under the influence of a combination of drugs.

NOTE: Tolerance to narcotics develops quickly making drug dependence very likely.

HEROIN
(COLOMBIAN)

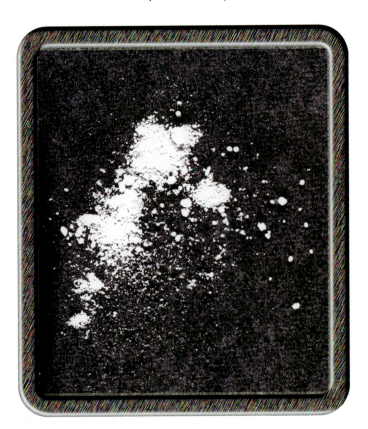

NARCOTICS

HEROIN
(COLOMBIAN)

Visual Description:
White powdered substance.

Methods of Use:
Ingested, Injected, Snorted

Duration of Effects:
Loaded: 4-6 Hours

Possible Effects:
Nystagmus - No
Pupils - Constricted
Pulse - Below Normal
Blood Pressure - Below Normal
Body Temperature - Normal/Below Normal
Non-Convergence - No

Depressed Reflexes
Droopy Eyelids (Ptosis)
Drowsiness
Dry Mouth
Euphoria
Fresh Puncture Marks
Impaired Divided Attention
Low, Raspy Voice
Nausea
Poor Muscle Coordination
Profuse Scratching
Vomiting

Overdose Symptoms:
Cold, Clammy Skin
Convulsions
Rapid, Weak pulse
Slow, Shallow Breathing
Coma
Death

Body Fluids Required For Testing: Urine (20cc) Blood is preferred.

NOTE: If you are unsure, it is advisable to take blood as the user may be under the influence of a combination of drugs.

NOTE: Tolerance to narcotics develops quickly making drug dependence very likely.

HEROIN
(PARAPHERNALIA)

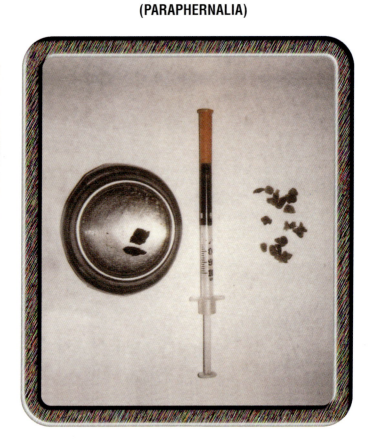

NARCOTICS

HEROIN
(PARAPHERNALIA)

EXPLANATION:

Powdered or Tar Heroin is placed in the "**cooker**", water is added, and solution is heated. A piece of cotton is added to act as a filter and the solution is drawn up into the needle. The arm is then "**tied-off**" with a belt, cord, or bandana to bulge the vein. The bulging of the vein is for easy injection and to cause the "**rush**" after the "**tie-off**" is released.

This injection process is the same for Cocaine and/or Methamphetamine injections except the drugs are not heated because they are water soluble. They are placed in the cooker and warm water is added.

NOTE: The "**cottons**" are kept. When the user does not have drugs, he will use the "**cottons**" to extract what ever small amount of Heroin is left in them. Cottons are considered drug residue and are not against the law to possess in some states.

HEROIN
(MEXICAN BROWN)

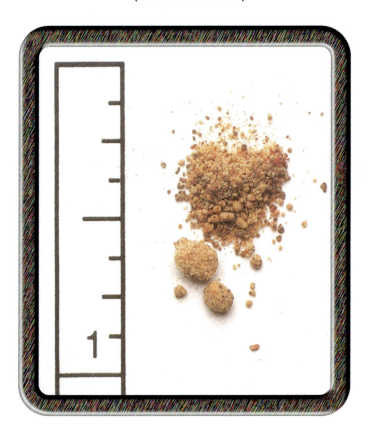

NARCOTICS

HEROIN
(MEXICAN BROWN)

Visual Description:
Powder that varies in color from white to dark brown.

Methods of Use:
Ingested, Injected, Smoked, Snorted

Duration of Effects:
Loaded: 4-6 Hours

Possible Effects:
Nystagmus - No
Pupils - Constricted
Pulse - Below Normal
Blood Pressure - Below Normal
Body Temperature - Normal/Below Normal
Non-Convergence - No

Depressed Reflexes
Droopy Eyelids (Ptosis)
Drowsiness
Dry Mouth
Euphoria
Profuse Scratching
Fresh Puncture Marks
Impaired Divided Attention
Low, Raspy Voice
Nausea
Poor Motor Coordination
Vomiting

Overdose Symptoms:
Cold, Clammy Skin
Convulsions
Rapid, Weak Pulse
Slow, Shallow Breathing
Coma
Death

Body Fluids Required For Testing: Urine (20cc) Blood is preferred.

NOTE: If you are unsure, it is advisable that blood is taken as the user may be under the influence of a combination of drugs.

NOTE: Tolerance to narcotics develops quickly making drug dependence very likely.

NARCOTICS

HEROIN
IN A BALLOON

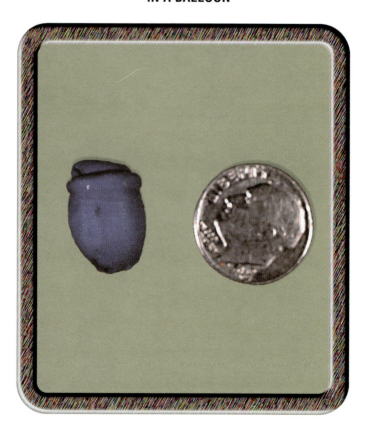

NARCOTICS

HEROIN
IN A BALLOON

EXPLANATION:

Frequently a toy balloon is used to package Mexican Brown Powdered Heroin. The balloon is used to enable the possessor to swallow the balloon if approached by authorities. It is later retrieved after defecation.

NARCOTICS

MEPERIDINE

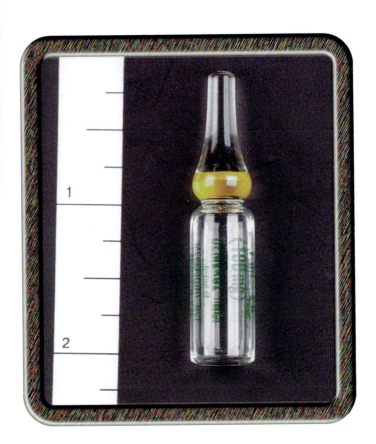

NARCOTICS

MEPERIDINE

Visual Description:
Liquid, Tablets, White Powder

Methods of Use:
Ingested, Injected, Snorted

Duration of Effects:
Loaded: 4-6 Hours

Possible Effects:
Nystagmus - No
Pupils - Constricted
Pulse - Below Normal
Blood Pressure - Below Normal
Body Temperature - Normal/Below Normal
Non-Convergence - No

Depressed Reflexes
Droopy Eyelids (Ptosis)
Drowsiness
Dry Mouth
Euphoria
Profuse Scratching
Fresh Puncture Marks
Impaired Divided Attention
Low, Raspy Voice
Nausea
Poor Motor Coordination
Vomiting

Overdose Symptoms:
Cold, Clammy Skin
Convulsions
Rapid, Weak Pulse
Slow, Shallow Breathing
Coma
Death

Body Fluids Required For Testing: Urine (20cc) Blood is preferred.

NOTE: If you are unsure, it is advisable to take blood as the user may be under the influence of a combination of drugs.

NOTE: Tolerance to narcotics develops quickly making drug dependence very likely.

METHADONE

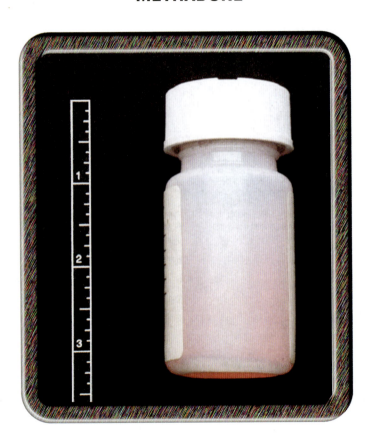

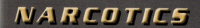

METHADONE

Visual Description:
Clear, Pink Liquid

Methods of Use:
Ingested, Injected

Duration of Effects:
Loaded: 12-24 Hours

Possible Effects:
Nystagmus - No
Pupils - Possibly Constricted
Pulse - Below Normal
Blood Pressure - Below Normal
Body Temperature - Normal/Below Normal
Non-Convergence - No

Depressed Reflexes
Droopy Eyelids (Ptosis)
Drowsiness
Dry Mouth
Euphoria
Fresh Puncture Marks
Impaired Divided Attention
Low, Raspy Voice
Nausea
Poor Motor Coordination
Vomiting

Overdose Symptoms:
Cold, Clammy Skin
Convulsions
Rapid, Weak Pulse
Slow, Shallow Breathing
Coma
Death

Body Fluids Required For Testing: Urine (20cc) Blood is preferred.

NOTE: If you are unsure, it is advisable that blood is taken as the user may be under the influence of a combination of drugs.

NOTE: When taken in proper doses, Methadone should not show any effects. It is used to keep the Heroin addict "well" and reduce the craving for Heroin.

METHADONE
(DOLOPHINE SULFATE)

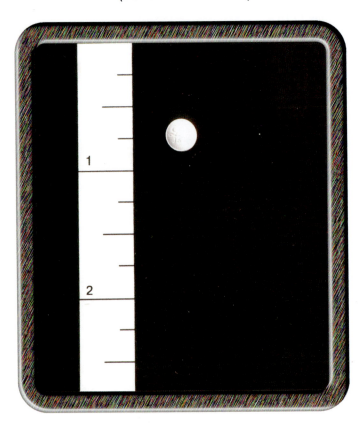

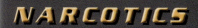

METHADONE
(DOLPHINE SULFATE)

Visual Description:
White Tablets

Methods of Use:
Ingested, Injected, Snorted

Duration of Effects:
Loaded: 12-24 Hours

Possible Effects:
Nystagmus - No
Pupils - Possibly Constricted
Pulse - Below Normal
Blood Pressure - Below Normal
Body Temperature - Normal/Below Normal
Non-Convergence - No

Depressed Reflexes
Droopy Eyelids (Ptosis)
Drowsiness
Dry Mouth
Euphoria
Fresh Puncture Marks

Impaired Divided Attention
Low, Raspy Voice
Nausea
Poor Motor Coordination
Vomiting

Overdose Symptoms:
Cold, Clammy Skin
Convulsions
Rapid, Weak Pulse
Slow, Shallow Breathing
Coma
Death

Body Fluids Required For Testing: Urine (20cc) Blood is preferred.

NOTE: If you are unsure, it is advisable that blood is taken as the user may be under the influence of a combination of drugs.

NOTE: When taken in proper doses, Methadone should not show any effects. It is used to keep the Heroin addict "well" and reduce the craving for Heroin.

NARCOTICS

METHADONE
FRONT SIDE OF IDENTIFICATION CARD

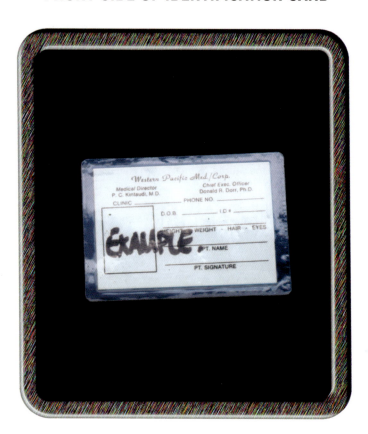

METHADONE
BACK SIDE OF IDENTIFICATION CARD

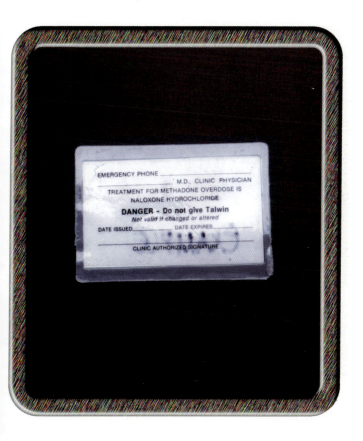

NARCOTICS

MORPHINE

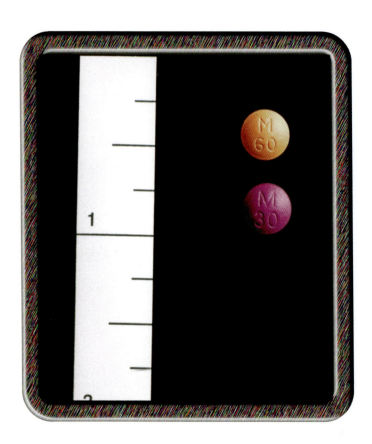

NARCOTICS

MORPHINE

Visual Description:
Tablets, Pink Liquid

Methods of Use:
Ingested, Injected, Snorted

Duration of Effects:
Loaded: 4-6 Hours

Possible Effects:
Nystagmus - No
Pupils - Constricted
Pulse - Below Normal
Blood Pressure - Below Normal
Body Temperature - Normal/Below Normal
Non-Convergence - No

Depressed Reflexes
Droopy Eyelids (Ptosis)
Drowsiness
Dry Mouth
Euphoria
Profuse Scratching
Fresh Puncture Marks
Impaired Divided Attention
Low, Raspy Voice
Nausea
Poor Motor Coordination
Vomiting

Overdose Symptoms:
Cold, Clammy Skin
Convulsions
Rapid, Weak Pulse
Slow, Shallow Breathing
Coma
Death

Body Fluids Required For Testing: Urine (20cc) Blood is preferred.

NOTE: If you are unsure, it is advisable to take blood as the user may be under the influence of a combination of drugs.

NOTE: Tolerance to narcotics develops quickly making drug dependence very likely.

NARCOTICS

OPIUM

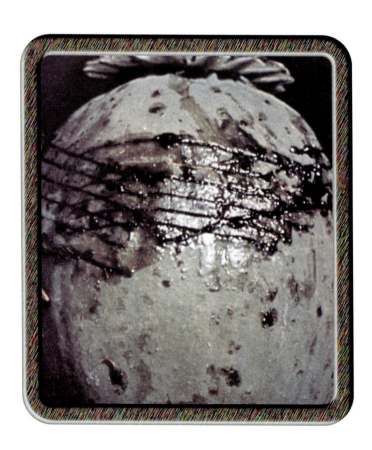

NARCOTICS

OPIUM

Visual Description:
Dark Brown Chunks, Powder

Methods of Use:
Injected, Ingested, Smoked, Snorted

Duration of Effects:
Loaded: 4-6 Hours

Possible Effects:
Nystagmus - No
Pupils - Constricted
Pulse - Below Normal
Blood Pressure - Below Normal
Body Temperature - Normal/Below Normal
Non-Convergence - No

Depressed Reflexes
Droopy Eyelids (Ptosis)
Drowsiness
Dry Mouth
Euphoria
Profuse Scratching
Fresh Puncture Marks
Impaired Divided Attention
Low, Raspy Voice
Nausea
Poor Motor Coordination
Vomiting

Overdose Symptoms:
Cold, Clammy Skin
Convulsions
Rapid, Weak Pulse
Slow, Shallow Breathing
Coma
Death

Body Fluids Required For Testing: Urine (20cc) Blood if preferred.

NOTE: If you are unsure, it is advisable to take blood as the user may be under the influence of a combination of drugs.

NOTE: Tolerance to narcotics develops quickly making drug dependence very likely.

NARCOTICS

PERCOCET

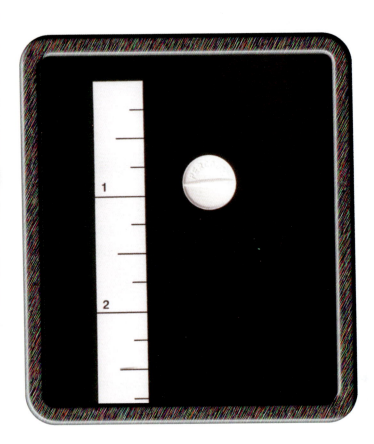

NARCOTICS

PERCOCET

Visual Description:
Tablets, Drops, Liquid

Methods of Use:
Ingested, Injected, Snorted

Duration of Effects:
Loaded: 4-6 Hours

Possible Effects:
Nystagmus - No
Pupils - Constricted
Pulse - Below Normal
Blood Pressure - Below Normal
Body Temperature - Normal/Below Normal
Non-Convergence - No

Depressed Reflexes
Droopy Eyelids (Ptosis)
Drowsiness
Dry Mouth
Euphoria
Profuse Scratching
Fresh Puncture Marks
Impaired Divided Attention
Low, Raspy Voice
Nausea
Poor Motor Coordination
Vomiting

Overdose Symptoms:
Cold, Clammy Skin
Convulsions
Rapid, Weak Pulse
Slow, Shallow Breathing
Coma
Death

Body Fluids Required For Testing: Urine (20cc) Blood if preferred.

NOTE: If you are unsure, it is advisable to take blood as the user may be under the influence of a combination of drugs.

NOTE: Tolerance to narcotics develops quickly making drug dependence very likely.

NARCOTICS

PERCODAN

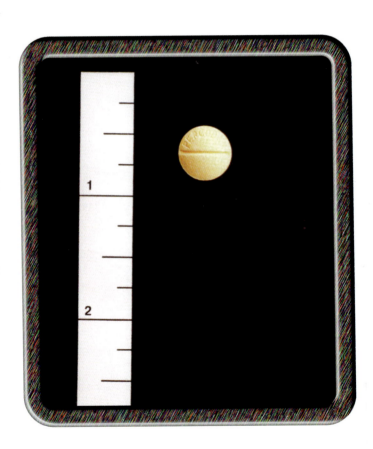

NARCOTICS

PERCODAN

Visual Description:
Tablets, Drops, Liquid

Methods of Use:
Ingested, Injected, Snorted

Duration of Effects:
Loaded: 4-6 Hours

Possible Effects:
Nystagmus - No
Pupils - Constricted
Pulse - Below Normal
Blood Pressure - Below Normal
Body Temperature - Normal/Below Normal
Non-Convergence - No

Depressed Reflexes
Droopy Eyelids (Ptosis)
Drowsiness
Dry Mouth
Euphoria
Profuse Scratching
Fresh Puncture Marks
Impaired Divided Attention
Low, Raspy Voice
Nausea
Poor Motor Coordination
Vomiting

Overdose Symptoms:
Cold, Clammy Skin
Convulsions
Rapid, Weak Pulse
Slow, Shallow Breathing
Coma
Death

Body Fluids Required For Testing: Urine (20cc) Blood if preferred.

NOTE: If you are unsure, it is advisable to take blood as the user may be under the influence of a combination of drugs.

NOTE: Tolerance to narcotics develops quickly making drug dependence very likely.

NARCOTICS

ADDITIONAL NARCOTICS

Darvocet
Darvon
Darvon-N
Fentanyl
Hycodan
Lomotil
Talwin
Tussionex

Visual Description:
Capsules, Liquid, Tablets

Methods of Use:
Ingested, Injected, Snorted

Duration of Effects:
Variable

Possible Effects:

- Depressed Reflexes
- Droopy Eyelids
- Drowsiness
- Dry Mouth
- Euphoria
- Coordination
- Vomiting
- Fresh Puncture Marks
- Impaired Divided Attention
- Low, Raspy Voice
- Nausea
- Poor Motor Skills
- Profuse Scratching

Body Fluids Required For Testing: Urine (20cc) Blood is preferred.

NOTE: If you are unsure, it is advisable to take blood as the user may be under the influence of a combination of drugs.

NOTE: Tolerance to narcotics develops quickly making drug dependency very likely.

NARCOTICS

PHENCYCLIDINE

P.C.P.

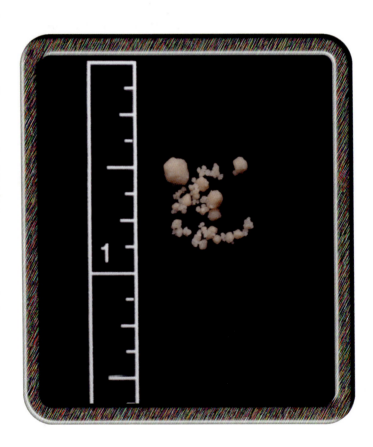

PHENCYCLIDINE

P.C.P.

Visual Description:
 Moist Brown Powder, White Crystalline Powder, Pills, Capsules

Methods of Use:
 Smoked, Ingested

Duration of Effects:
 Onset: 1-5 Minutes   Loaded: 4-6 Hours
 Peak: 15-30 Minutes   Normal: Variable

Possible Effects:
 Nystagmus - Yes (Vertical & Horizontal)
 Pupils - Near Normal
 Pulse - Elevated
 Blood Pressure - Elevated
 Body Temperature - Elevated
 Non-Convergence - Yes

 Agitation
 Aggressive
 Blank Stare
 Cyclic Behavior
 Disoriented
 High Pain Threshold
 Incomplete Verbal Response
 Muscle Rigidity
 Non-Communicative
 Odor of Substance
 Perspiring
 Repetitive Speech
 Warm to the Touch

Overdose Symptoms:
 Bizarre Behavior
 Long, Intense Trips
 Psychosis
 Violence
 Death

Body Fluids Required For Testing: Blood

PHENCYCLIDINE

P.C.P.
(LIQUID)

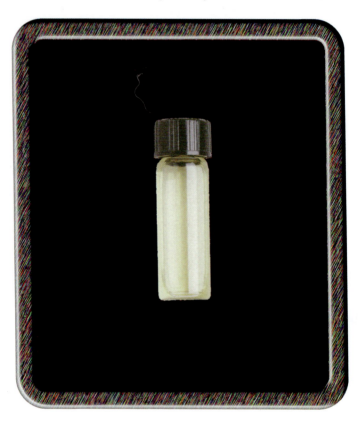

PHENCYCLIDINE

P.C.P.
(LIQUID)

Visual Description:
Clear Yellow Liquid

Methods of Use:
Ingested, Smoked,

Duration of Effects:
Onset: 1-5 Minutes   Loaded: 4-6 Hours
Peak: 15-30 Minutes   Normal: Variable

Possible Effects:
Nystagmus - Yes (Vertical & Horizontal)
Pupils - Near Normal
Pulse - Elevated
Blood Pressure - Elevated
Body Temperature - Elevated
Non-Convergence - Yes

Agitation Muscle Rigidity   Muscle Rigidity
Aggressive   Non-Communicative
Blank Stare   Odor of Substance
Cyclic Behavior   Perspiring
Disoriented   Repetitive Speech
High Pain Threshold   Warm to the Touch
Incomplete Verbal Response

Overdose Symptoms:
Bizarre Behavior
Long, Intense Trips
Psychosis
Violence
Death

Body Fluids Required For Testing: Blood

PSYCHEDELIC AMPHETAMINE

ECSTASY
(XTC)

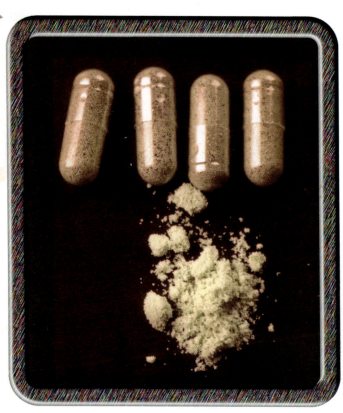

PSYCHEDELIC AMPHETAMINE

ECSTASY
(XTC)

Visual Description:
Brown Crystalline Powder

Methods of Use:
Ingested, Injected

Duration of Effects:
Variable

Possible Effects:
- **Nystagmus** - No
- **Pupils** - Dilated
- **Pulse** - Elevated
- **Blood Pressure** - Elevated
- **Body Temperature** - Elevated
- **Non-Convergence** - No

Anxiety
Blurred Vision
Chills or Sweating
Depression
Faintness
Fresh Puncture Marks
Hallucinations
Hyperactive
Impaired Divided Attention
Lack of Inhibitions
Paranoia

Overdose Symptoms:
Bizarre Behavior
Long, Intense Trips
Psychosis
Violence
Death

Body Fluids Required For Testing: Blood

NOTE: Analogs may be several hundred times stronger than the drugs they were designed to imitate. Therefore, the effect may be much more severe or intense.

PSYCHEDELIC AMPHETAMINE

ECSTASY
(XTC)

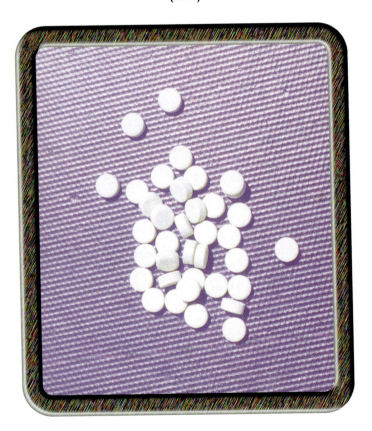

PSYCHEDELIC AMPHETAMINE

ECSTASY
(XTC)

Visual Description:
Tablets in many different colors

Methods of Use:
Ingested, Injected, Snorted

Duration of Effects:
Variable

Possible Effects:
- **Nystagmus -** No
- **Pupils -** Dilated
- **Pulse -** Elevated
- **Blood Pressure -** Elevated
- **Body Temperature -** Elevated
- **Non-Convergence -** No

Anxiety
Blurred Vision
Chills or Sweating
Depression
Faintness
Fresh Puncture Marks
Hallucinations
Hyperactive
Impaired Divided Attention
Lack of Inhibitions
Paranoia

Overdose Symptoms:
Bizarre Behavior
Long, Intense Trips
Psychosis
Violence
Death

Body Fluids Required For Testing: Blood

NOTE: Analogs may be several hundred times stronger than the drugs they were designed to imitate. Therefore, the effect may be much more severe or intense.

STIMULANTS

AMPHETAMINES

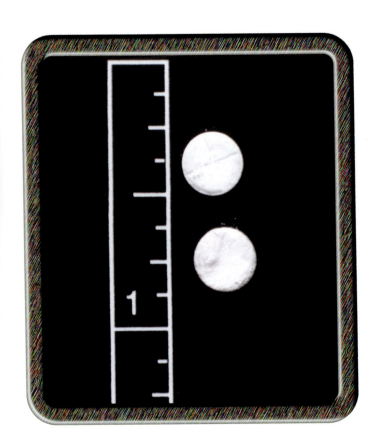

STIMULANTS

AMPHETAMINES

Visual Description:
Capsules, Crystal, Pills, Double Scored Tablets, Powder, Solid Rock

Methods of Use:
Ingested, Injected, Smoked, Snorted

Duration of Effects:
Onset: 30-40 Seconds   Loaded: 4-8 Hours

Possible Effects:
Nystagmus - No
Pupils - Dilated
Pulse - Elevated
Blood Pressure - Elevated
Body Temperature - Elevated
Non-Convergence - No

- Anxiety
- Body Tremors
- Decreased Appetite
- Dizziness
- Dry Mouth
- Euphoria
- Excitation
- Fresh Puncture Marks
- Grinding Teeth (Bruxism)
- Hallucinations
- Headaches
- Impaired Divided Attention
- Increased Alertness
- Insomnia
- Loss of Coordination
- Restlessness
- Sweating

Overdose Symptoms:
- Agitation
- Convulsions
- Death

Body Fluids Required For Testing: Blood

NOTE: An Amphetamine injection creates a sudden rise in blood pressure that can cause a stroke, very high fever or heart attack. Prolonged use can cause hallucinations, delusions, and paranoia.

STIMULANTS

BIPHETAMINES

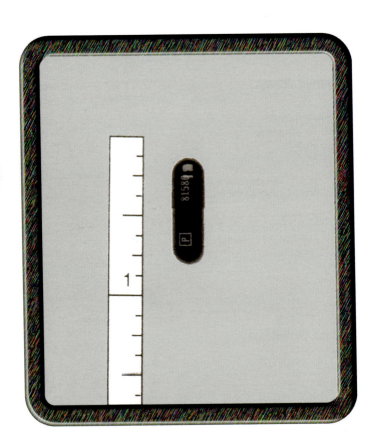

STIMULANTS

BIPHETAMINES

Visual Description:
Capsules, Powder

Methods of Use:
Ingested, Injected, Snorted

Duration of Effects:
Onset: 30-40 Seconds   Loaded: 4-8 Hours

Possible Effects:
- **Nystagmus** - No
- **Pupils** - Dilated
- **Pulse** - Elevated
- **Blood Pressure** - Elevated
- **Body Temperature** - Elevated
- **Non-Convergence** - No

Anxiety	Hallucinations
Body Tremors	Headaches
Decreased Appetite	Impaired Divided Attention
Dizziness	Increased Alertness
Dry Mouth	Insomnia
Euphoria	Loss of Coordination
Excitation	Restlessness
Fresh Puncture Marks	Sweating
Grinding Teeth (Bruxism)	

Overdose Symptoms:
- Agitation
- Convulsions
- Death

Body Fluids Required For Testing: Blood

NOTE: An Amphetamine injection creates a sudden rise in blood pressure that can cause a stroke, very high fever or heart attack. Prolonged use can cause hallucinations, delusions, and paranoia.

STIMULANTS

COCAINE
(CRACK OR FREEBASE)

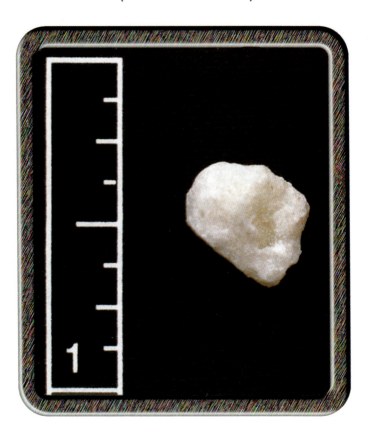

STIMULANTS

COCAINE
(CRACK OR FREEBASE)

Visual Description:
Light brown, beige or white crystalline rocks often packaged in small vials or small zip-lock plastic bags.

Methods of Use:
Smoked

Duration of Effects:
Onset: 8-30 Seconds   Loaded: 15-30 Minutes
Peak: 5-15 Minutes   Normal: 60-90 Minutes

Possible Effects:
Nystagmus - No
Pupils - Dilated
Pulse - Elevated
Blood Pressure - Elevated
Body Temperature - Elevated
Non-Convergence - No

Anxiety
Body Tremors
Decreased Appetite
Dizziness
Dry Mouth
Euphoria
Excitation
Grinding Teeth (Bruxism)
Hallucinations

Hacking Cough
Headaches
Impaired Divided Attention
Increased Alertness
Insomnia
Loss of Coordination
Restlessness
Sweating

Overdose Symptoms:
Agitation
Convulsions
Death

Body Fluids Required For Testing: Blood

NOTE: Crack or Freebase rock is very addictive.

STIMULANTS

COCAINE
(CRACK/FREEBASE PARAPHERNALIA)

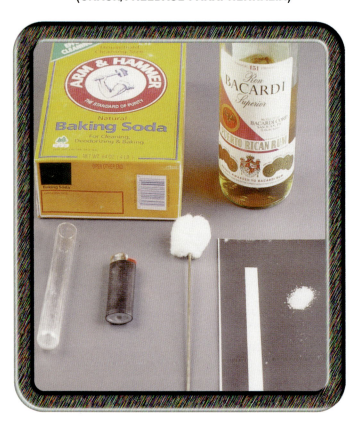

STIMULANTS

COCAINE
(CRACK/FREEBASE PARAPHERNALIA)

EXPLANATION:

A mixture of Cocaine and baking soda is put into the cooker, mixed with water and heated. The solution will go from a solid, to a liquid, to a transparent oil that will collect at the bottom of the cooker. (Heat Source: Cotton ball soaked in rum.) The Cocaine is cooled in water and the oil forms a rock. The rock is placed in a pipe and smoked. (The rock does not burn, but vaporizes.) The vapors are inhaled.

STIMULANTS

COCAINE
(POWDER)

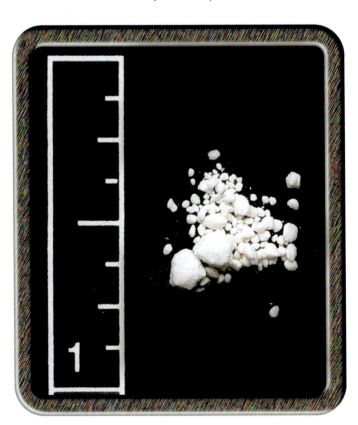

STIMULANTS

COCAINE
(POWDER)

Visual Description:
White Crystalline Powder (often diluted with other ingredients).

Methods of Use:
Injected, Snorted

Duration of Effects:
Onset: 15-30 Seconds
Peak: 5-15 Minutes
Loaded: 15-20 Minutes
Normal: 60-90 Minutes

Possible Effects:
Nystagmus - No
Pupils - Dilated
Pulse - Elevated
Blood Pressure - Elevated
Body Temperature - Elevated
Non-Convergence - No

- Anxiety
- Body Tremors
- Impaired Divided Attention
- Decreased Appetite
- Dizziness
- Euphoria
- Excitation
- Running/Red/Bleeding Nose
- Fresh Puncture Marks
- Grinding Teeth (Bruxism)
- Headaches
- Hallucinations
- Excitation
- Increased Alertness
- Insomnia
- Loss of Coordination
- Restlessness
- Sweating
- Talkative
- Dry Mouth

Overdose Symptoms:
Agitation
Convulsions
Death

Body Fluids Required For Testing: Blood

NOTE: Occasional use of Cocaine can cause a stuffy or bloody nose, while long-term use may result in the ulceration of the mucous membranes of the nose or complete perforation of the nasal septum.

STIMULANTS

COCAINE
(POWDER-PARAPHERNALIA)

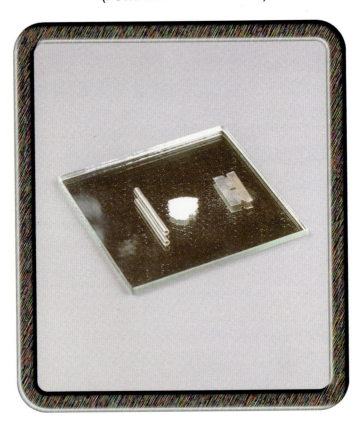

STIMULANTS

COCAINE
(POWDER-PARAPHERNALIA)

EXPLANATION:

Powdered Cocaine is placed on a mirror or piece of glass (flat, non-porous surface). It is then chopped into a fine powder with a razor blade or credit card. The Cocaine is then spread into thin lines, and the lines are then snorted through a tube.

STIMULANTS

METHAMPHETAMINE
(ICE)

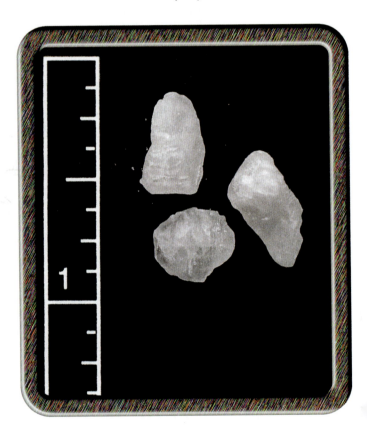

STIMULANTS

METHAMPHETAMINE
(ICE)

Visual Description:
White Crystalline Rock

Methods of Use:
Smoked

Duration of Effects:
Onset: 8-30 Seconds
Loaded: 12-20 Hours

Possible Effects:
Nystagmus - No
Pupils - Dilated
Pulse - Elevated
Blood Pressure - Elevated
Body Temperature - Elevated
Non-Convergence - No

Anxiety
Blurred Vision
Body Tremors
Chills or Sweating
Depression
Euphoria
Excitation
Faintness
Gait Ataxia
Grinding of Teeth (Bruxism)
Hallucinations
Increased Alertness
Insomnia
Restlessness

Overdose Symptoms:
Bizarre Behavior
Long, Intense Trips
Psychosis
Violence
Coma
Death

Body Fluids Required For Testing: Blood

NOTE: The drug ICE is a smokable form of crystal methamphetamine.

STIMULANTS

METHAMPHETAMINE
(CRANK OR SPEED)

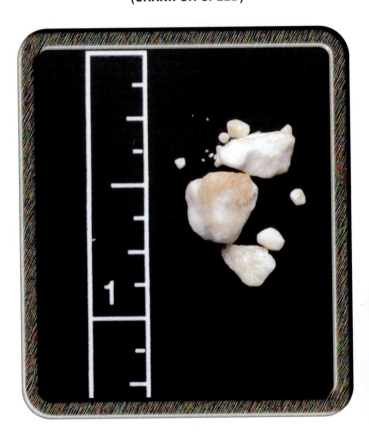

STIMULANTS

METHAMPHETAMINE
(CRANK OR SPEED)

Visual Description:
Beige Powder, White Crystalline Rock, White Powder

Methods of Use:
Injected, Smoked, Snorted

Duration of Effects:
Onset: 30-40 Seconds   Loaded: 4-8 Hours

Possible Effects:
- **Nystagmus -** No
- **Pupils -** Dilated
- **Pulse -** Elevated
- **Blood Pressure -** Elevated
- **Body Temperature -** Elevated
- **Non-Convergence -** No

- Anxiety
- Body Tremors
- Decreased Appetite
- Dizziness
- Dry Mouth
- Euphoria
- Excitation
- Fresh Puncture Marks
- Grinding Teeth (Bruxism)
- Hallucinations
- Impaired Divided Attention
- Increased Alertness
- Insomnia
- Loss of Coordination
- Restlessness
- Sweating

Overdose Symptoms:
- Agitation
- Convulsions
- Hallucinations
- Psychosis
- Coma
- Death

Body Fluids Required For Testing: Blood

STIMULANTS

METHCATHINONE

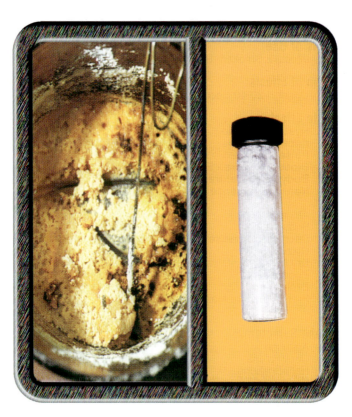

RAW   **PURE**

STIMULANTS

METHCATHINONE

Visual Description:
White Crystalline Powder

Methods of Use:
Injected, Snorted

Duration of Effects:
Loaded from 30 minutes to 24 hours depending on dosage taken.

Possible Effects:
Nystagmus - No
Pupils - Dilated
Pulse - Elevated
Blood Pressure - Elevated
Body Temperature - Elevated
Non-Convergence - No

- Anxiety
- Body Tremors
- Decreased Appetite
- Dizziness
- Dilusions
- Dry Mouth
- Euphoria
- Excitation
- Fresh Puncture Marks
- Grinding Teeth (Bruxism)
- Hallucinations
- Headaches
- Impaired Divided Attention
- Increased Alertness
- Insomnia
- Loss of Coordination
- Restlessness
- Sweating

Overdose Symptoms:
- Agitation
- Convulsions
- Hallucinations
- Psychosis
- Coma
- Death

Body Fluids Required For Testing: Blood
NOTE: Tolerance builds quickly.

STIMULANTS

ADDITIONAL STIMULANTS
Cathinone
Cylert
Didrex
Ionamin
Preludin
Ritalin

Methods of Use:
Ingested, Injected

Duration of Effects:
Variable

Possible Effects:
Anxiety
Body Tremors
Dry Mouth
Euphoria
Excitation
Fresh Puncture Marks
Grinding Teeth (Bruxism)
Increased Alertness
Insomnia
Restlessness

Overdose Symptoms:
Agitation
Convulsions
Hallucinations
High Body Temperature
Coma
Death

Body Fluids Required For Testing: Blood

PARAPHERNALIA IDENTIFICATION & DESCRIPTIONS

ASSORTED SMOKING PARAPHERNALIA

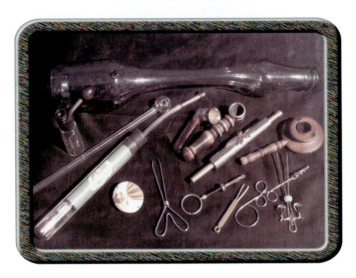

PARAPHERNALIA

BINDLE

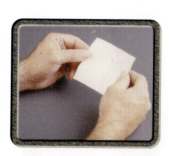

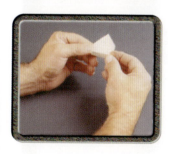

EXPLANATION:
A bindle is a small piece of paper, folded like an envelope to form a pocket, used to hold a personal amount of a drug.

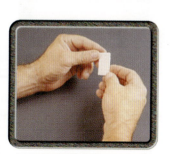

PARAPHERNALIA

COCAINE SIFTER

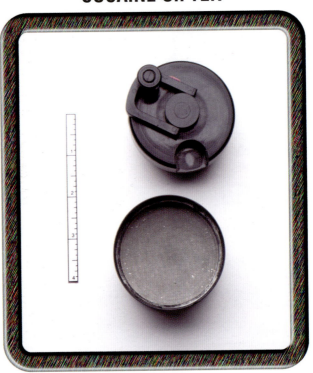

METHODS OF USE:
The drug is placed in the top compartment. The lid is screwed on and the handle is turned (forcing the powder through the screen), making the powder a very fine texture for snorting.

PARAPHERNALIA

COPPER SCOURING PADS

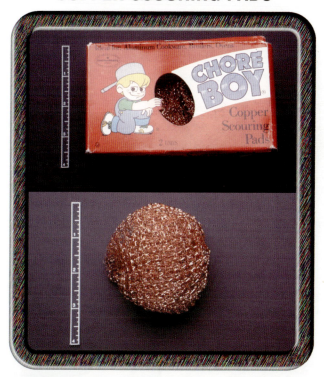

METHODS OF USE:
Small, round pieces of these pads are placed in bowls of Freebase Pipes. The **"rock"** is then placed on top of the pad and lit. The metal fibers of the pad hold the melting **"rock"** and keep it hot. The most popular brand of copper pad is **"Chore Boy"**. Very fine steel wool or **"Brillo Pads"** are also used.

PARAPHERNALIA

DRUG LAB

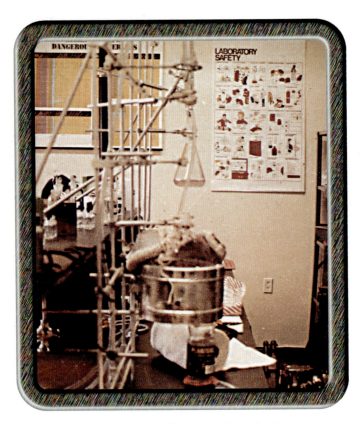

Methamphetamine Lab

PARAPHERNALIA

FREEBASE SMOKING PIPE

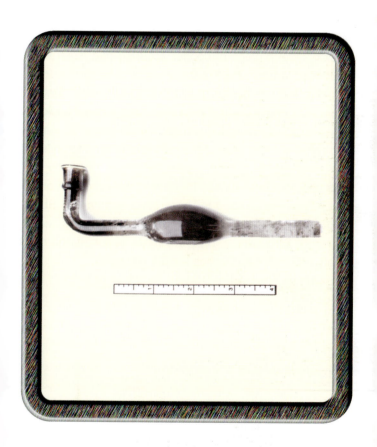

PARAPHERNALIA

FREEBASE SMOKING PIPE

METHODS OF USE:

After placing a piece of copper scouring pad, steel wool or Brillo Pad in bowl, the Freebase Rock is placed on top and lit. The rock will begin to vaporize and melt. Since the vapors are heavier than the air, they drop into the neck of the pipe and are drawn into the lungs. Some pipes have a bulge or chamber in the neck of the pipe that is used to collect the vapor and accumulate it before it is inhaled into the lungs. This chamber is also used for cooling the vapor. (A glass or metal tube is also used.) These tubes are called **"Straight Shooters."** Automotive radio antennas are also used as **"Straight Shooters."** They are easily obtained and can be easily dropped if authorities should approach.

See WASHBACK METHODS on Page 161.

PARAPHERNALIA

HEROIN
(USED "COTTONS", COOKER & LOADED SYRINGE)

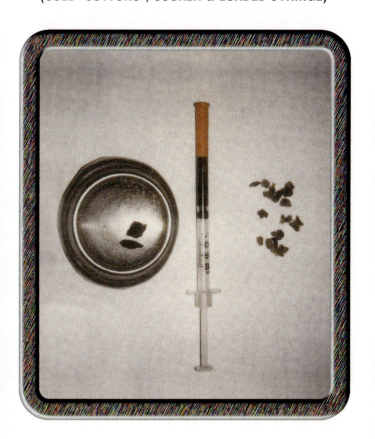

Paraphernalia

HEROIN
(CONTAINED IN A TOY BALLOON)

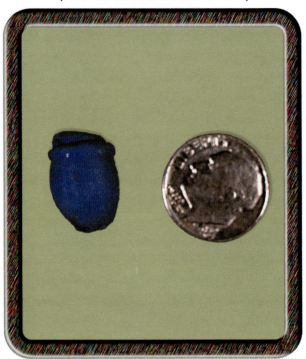

METHODS OF USE:

Frequently a toy balloon is used to package Mexican Powdered Heroin. The balloon is used to enable the possessor to swallow the balloon if approached by authorities. It is later retrieved after defecation.

PARAPHERNALIA

MARIJUANA ROACH CLIPS

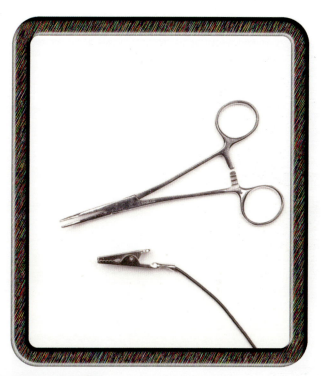

METHODS OF USE:
These are the commonly used "**Roach Clips**". They are used to hold the last bit of a burning Marijuana cigarette.

PARAPHERNALIA

METHAMPHETAMINE (ICE) SMOKING PIPE

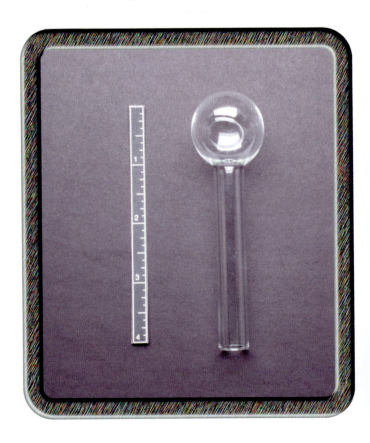

PARAPHERNALIA

METHAMPHETAMINE (ICE) SMOKING PIPE

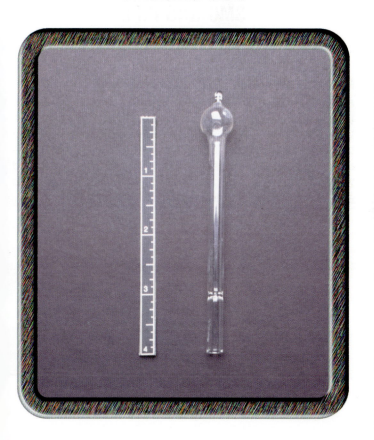

PARAPHERNALIA

METHAMPHETAMINE (ICE) SMOKING PIPE

METHODS OF USE:
A piece of **ICE** is placed inside the round portion of the pipe. It is then heated from beneath which causes vapors that are then drawn into the lungs. These pipes have a small hole at the top of the round chamber. When the drug is heated, the user places a finger over the hole. The finger is removed when the vapor is drawn into the lungs. The user often has a round burn mark on the finger.

PARAPHERNALIA

METHAMPHETAMINE (ICE) SMOKING PIPE

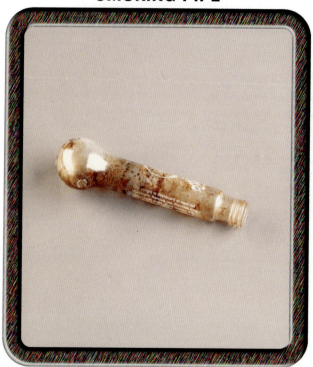

EXPLANATION:

A commercial automobile air freshener is emptied. The end of the tube is heated and then blown into which creates a bulge at the end. A hole is poked through the bulging end with a hot needle.

PARAPHERNALIA

METHAMPHETAMINE (ICE) SMOKING PIPE
(MADE FROM LIGHT BULBS)

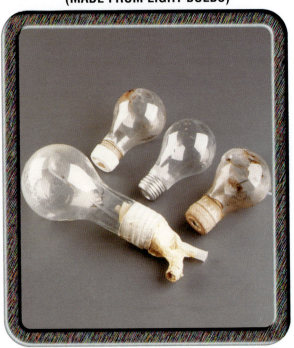

METHODS OF USE:
The end of the light bulb is cut off and the insides discarded. A hole is then poked through the rounded end with a hot needle.

PARAPHERNALIA

METHAMPHETAMINE (ICE) ASSORTED SMOKING PIPES
(HOMEMADE & COMMERCIAL)

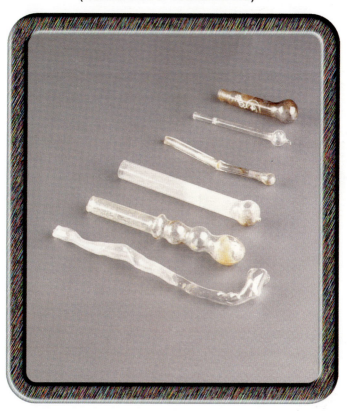

PARAPHERNALIA

SCALES
(POCKET DRUG-WEIGHING SCALE)

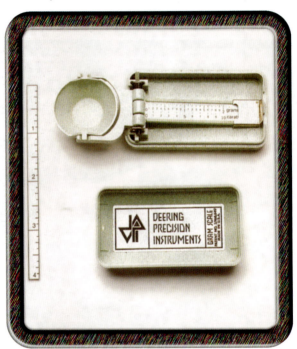

METHODS OF USE:

These scales are often used by **"Pookct Dealers."** (These are dealers who sell in small quantities, such as a gram.) The scale is assembled and the amount desired is set on the slide arm. The drug is then added to the bowl until the arm is level.

PARAPHERNALIA

SCALES
(COMMON DRUG-WEIGHING SCALE)

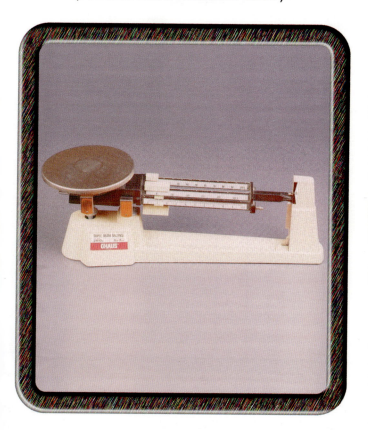

PARAPHERNALIA

SNORTING SPOON

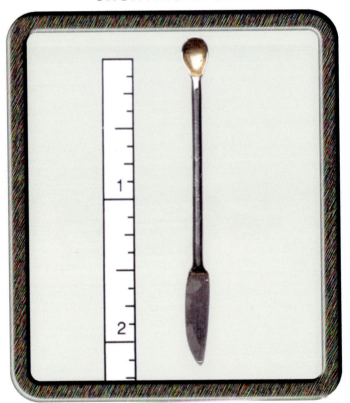

METHODS OF USE:

The desired amount of the drug is placed in the bowl of the spoon. One nostril is closed while the other nostril is used to snort the drug from the spoon.

PARAPHERNALIA

SNORTING TUBES

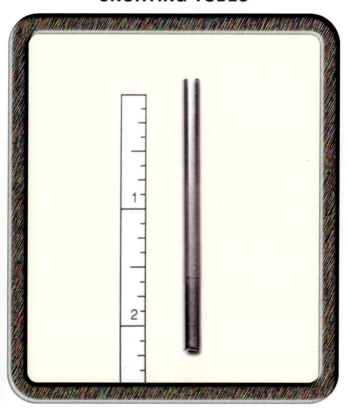

PARAPHERNALIA

SNORTING TUBES

METHODS OF USE:
The desired amount of the drug is placed on a smooth surface such as a piece of glass or mirror. A razor blade or a straight edge, such as a credit card, is used to chop the drug into fine particles. A **"line"** is then made with the substance. The tube is placed into one nostril while the other nostril is closed. The drug is then snorted through the tube.

PARAPHERNALIA

SNORTING VIAL

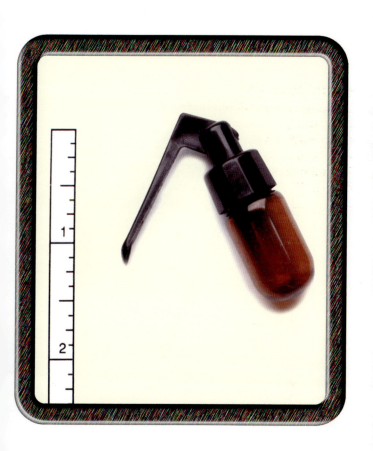

PARAPHERNALIA

SNORTING VIAL

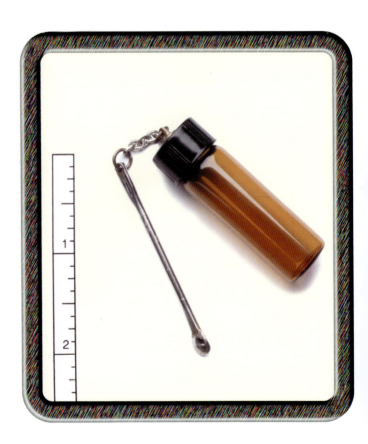

PARAPHERNALIA

SNORTING VIAL

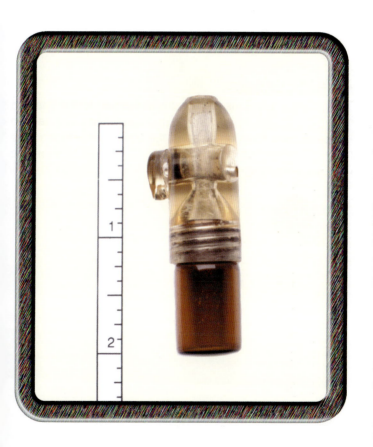

PARAPHERNALIA

SNORTING VIAL

METHODS OF USE:
The snorting vile is used in a similar fashion to the snorting spoon as the vile usually has a spoon attached. The desired amount of the drug is placed in the bowl of the spoon, one nostril is closed while the other nostril is used to snort the drug from the spoon.

PARAPHERNALIA

STASH CANS

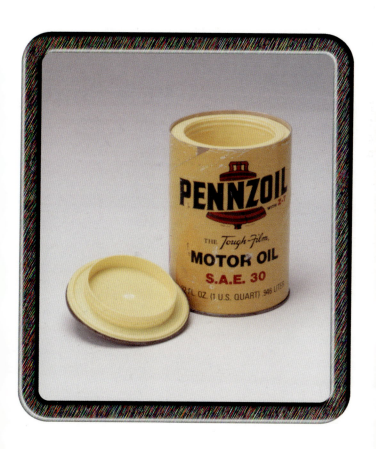

PARAPHERNALIA

STASH CANS

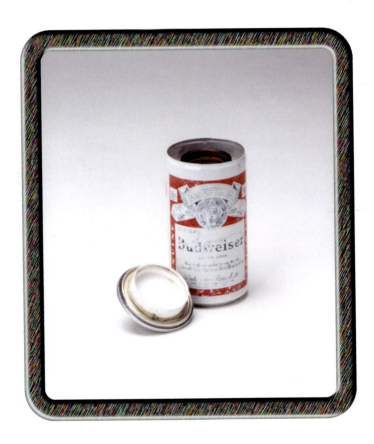

PARAPHERNALIA

STASH CANS

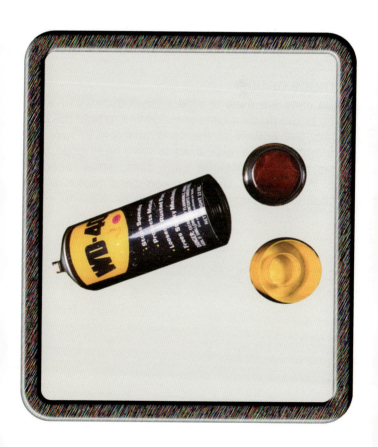

PARAPHERNALIA

STASH CANS

METHODS OF USE:
These cans are used to hide a small quantity of a drug. Name brand product cans are modified to hold the drugs. Usually the bottom of the cans unscrew to reveal the compartment. (Reverse threads have been used lately.) Stash cans may include beer cans, spray deodorant cans, WD-40 cans, shaving cream cans, motor oil cans, and countless other products.

PARAPHERNALIA

WASHBACK METHODS

As Cocaine vapors travel the length of the pipe, some of the vapors dry and adhere to the sides of the pipe. The following processes are popular street methods for retrieving usable Cocaine that is trapped inside the Freebase Pipe.

WET WASH METHOD:
A small amount of 151 rum is put into the mouthpiece of the pipe and the inside is washed out. The rum is then poured on a mirror or a piece of glass, lit, and some of the rum is burned off. A piece of copper pad, Brillo pad or steel wool is rubbed around to soak up what is left after burning. The pad is then placed in the pipe, lit, and the vapors drawn into the lungs.

DRY WASH METHOD:
A small amount of 151 rum is put into the mouthpiece of the pipe and the inside washed out. The rum is then poured on a mirror or piece of glass, lit, and burned until it is completely dry. What is left on the glass or mirror is usable Cocaine. This is then scrapped off the glass, placed in the pipe and smoked. The Dry Wash Method is the most popular.

NOTE: The Washback Methods are primarily used with a Freebase Cocaine Pipe, but may also be used with an ICE or Methamphetamine Pipe.

NEEDLE INJECTIONS/ PUNCTURE WOUNDS

NEEDLE INJECTIONS/ PUNCTURE WOUNDS

STERILE INJECTIONS

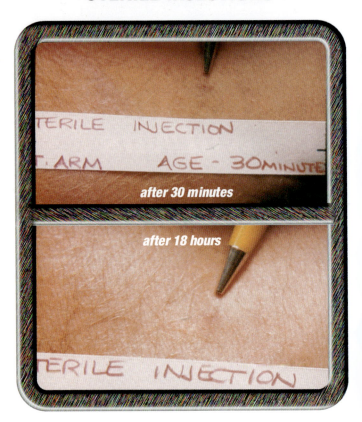

after 30 minutes

after 18 hours

NEEDLE INJECTIONS/ PUNCTURE WOUNDS

UNSTERILE INJECTIONS

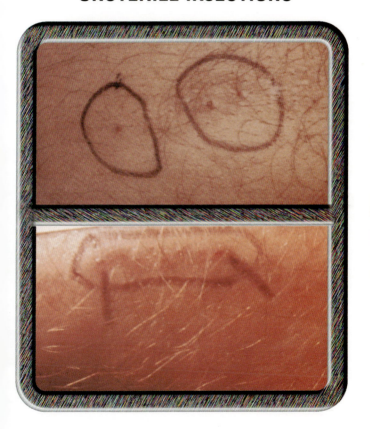

WEIGHTS & MEASURES

WEIGHTS & MEASURES

EQUIVALENT WEIGHTS AND MEASURES

DRY MEASURES:

1 Microgram (mcg.)	=	1/1000 of a Milligram (mg)
1000 Micrograms (mcg.)	=	1 Milligram (mg.)
1000 grams	=	1 Kilogram (kilo.)
1 Kilogram (kilo.)	=	2.2 Pounds (lbs.)
1 Gram (g.)	=	15.43 Grains (gr.)
28.35 grams (g.)	=	1 Ounce (oz.)
453.6 Grams (g.)	=	1 Pound (lb.)
1 Grain (gr.)	=	65 Milligrams (mg.)
1 Grain (gr.)	=	.065 Grams (g.)
1 Ounce (oz.)	=	437.5 Grains (gr.)
1 Ounce (oz.)	=	28.35 grams (g.)
1 Ounce (oz.)	=	28,350 Milligrams (mg.)
1 Ounce (oz.)	=	6 Tablespoons (tbls.) approx.
1 Pound (lb.)	=	7,000 Grains (gr.)
1 Pound (lb.)	=	16 Ounces (oz.)
1 Pound (lb.)	=	453 Grams (g.)
1 Ton	=	2,000 (lbs.)

DRUG TESTING

DRUG TESTING

PUPIL/LIGHT ACCOMMODATION TEST:

The purpose of this series of tests is to examine the reaction, or lack of reaction, to the presence and absence of light. Use a pen light and a Pupilometer. (Average pupil size is 3.0 to 6.5 millimeters.)

AVAILABLE LIGHT:

Using whatever light is available at the time of the test, use a Pupilometer to check the size of both pupils. Always check the left pupil first (to keep the test standardized and systematic) and note the size of each pupil separately. To do this, place the Pupilometer along the temple side of the eye. Locate the circle that best matches the size of the pupil and note that size. (Do not cover any portion of the eye with the Pupilometer during this test.)

CLOSE TO TOTAL DARKNESS:

Expose the subject's eyes to a minimum of 90 seconds of uninterrupted, total darkness. Next, place the pad of the index finger over the lens of the pen light. (This will result in a red light.) Place the Pupilometer on the temple side of the eye and shine the red light into the eye. Measure the size of the pupil, doing the left eye first (to keep the test standardized and systematic), then note the size of each pupil separately.

INDIRECT LIGHT:

Using the white light of the pen light, illuminate the temple about 6 inches away from the side of the head. Bring inner beam of light forward until it shines across the front of eyeball,

DRUG TESTING (con't)

creating a shadow or silhouette on the side of the nose halfway between the corner of the eye and the bridge of the nose. Place Pupilometer beside the left eye first (to standardize test) and measure the size of the pupil of each eye separately. (Do not shade the light with the Pupilometer.)

DIRECT LIGHT:

Shine the inner beam of the pen light directly into the eye. Position the beam of light between the eyebrows and the top of the cheekbone. Hold the light in this position for one minute. Measure the size of the pupil of the left eye first (to standardize test) with the Pupilometer. Note the measurement of each pupil separately.

HORIZONTAL NYSTAGMUS TEST

SMOOTH PURSUIT:

While the subject is looking straight ahead, place a stimulus (index finger) 15 inches in front of the tip of the nose and even with the eyebrows. Move the stimulus (index finger) to the subject's left about 45 degrees watching for an involuntary jerking of the eyes. Proceed to move the stimulus (index finger) to the right eye and repeat procedure. Do this twice with each eye. When moving the stimulus (index finger) to the left, check the left eye. When moving the stimulus (index finger) to the right, check the right eye. Move the stimulus (index finger) straight across in front of the subject's face.

HORIZONTAL NYSTAGMUS TEST (con't)

MAXIMUM DEVIATION:
Administer this test in the exact same manner as the Smooth Pursuit Test except at 45 degrees, hold the stimulus (index finger) still for 5 seconds. Look for involuntary jerking of the eye.
NOTE: Some people have nystagmus naturally.

ANGLE OF ONSET
Begin with the stimulus in the same manner as in smooth pursuit. Move outward from the tip of the nose towards the subject's left. When nystagmus is first observed stop, you are trying to determine the angle of onset in degrees. At 15 inches from the subjects face, the end of the left shoulder is approximately 45 degrees. The equation is, 50 - angle of onset = blood alcohol concentration.
EXAMPLE: A 45 degree angle of onset equals a .05 B.A.C.

VERTICAL NYSTAGMUS TEST
With the subject looking straight ahead, place the stimulus (index finger) 15 inches out from the tip of the nose. Move stimulus (index finger) upward level with the top of the head and hold for 5 seconds, then down to the tip of the nose. Do this test at least twice looking at each eye once. Record your results.
NOTE: Vertical Nystagmus is when the eyeballs jerk vertically (up and down).

DRUG TESTING

NON-CONVERGENCE TEST

When the subject is looking straight ahead, place the stimulus (index finger) 15 inches in front of the tip of the nose. First move the stimulus in front of the face counter clockwise. The circles should not be larger than the subject's face.

When you are sure the subject is following the stimulus with his eyes, bring the stimulus (index finger) to the nose and touch the bridge of the nose. Tell the subject to watch the stimulus (index finger) on the bridge of the nose for at least 5 seconds. Look for either or both eyes drifting outward, not being able to focus inward on the nose.

NOTE: Non-convergence can be natural in some individuals.

DRUG TESTING

STANDARD FIELD SOBRIETY TESTS

The following is an explanation of the four standardized field sobriety tests. Please keep in mind:

1. These tests should be used for ALL drug influence situations, not just for alcohol intoxication.

2. Give clear instructions to the subject and be sure they understand what is required of them before they begin each test.

3. Conduct each test on a flat surface that is well-lit and void of any obstructions.

4. Discontinue any test if the subject is in any danger of injury.

5. Take complete notes as you administer each test.

6. These tests should be given in the same order and instructed in the same way each time to standardize the tests.

DRUG TESTING

FIELD SOBRIETY TESTS

RHOMBERG 30 SECOND ESTIMATION OF TIME: During the explanation and demonstration of this test, have the subject stand upright with heels and toes together and their hands at their sides. This is the "Rhomberg Position."

TEST: In the **"Rhomberg Position,"** have the subject tilt his head back and close his eyes. When you say begin, have the subject estimate 30 seconds. (This should be done silently.) When the subject believes the 30 seconds are finished, he should open his eyes and bring his head forward. This indicates the end of the test. If the subject has not completed the test in 90 seconds, discontinue the test.

NOTES:

1. Drugs that speed up the body will cause a short estimation of time (Cocaine, amphetamines, etc.), and the drugs that slow the system down will cause a long estimation of time (depressants, narcotics, alcohol, etc.).

2. Be aware of the actual time during the test. Note any body movements such as swaying, body tremors, muscle rigidity, etc.

3. Make sure the subject performs the test as instructed.

DRUG TESTING

WALK AND TURN

During the explanation and demonstration, have the subject place his right foot on the line he will be walking on. Then have him place the toes of his left foot against the heel of his right foot. Standing flat on the ground with both feet pointing in the same direction, stand up straight with both arms at his side.

TEST: Instruct the subject to walk nine steps up the line, turn around and walk nine steps back. (Each step should be heel to toe.) The subject will look down at his feet and count each step out loud. At the end of the first nine steps, the subject will turn. (The turn will be a three-point pivot, keeping the front foot in its place and using the balls of this foot to pivot.) With the back foot, push three times around to face the opposite direction. Walk back nine steps in the same manner. If at any time the subject falls off the line, he is to regain his balance and continue to walk and count off his steps where he left off. Discontinue test if subject is in danger of injury.

NOTES:

1. Note any difficulties balancing.

2. Note if the subject uses his arms or any other object for balance.

3. Be sure he touches heel to toe as instructed.

4. Make sure the turn is done as instructed.

5. The counting of steps should be loud enough to be heard.

6. Make sure the subject performs the test as instructed.

ONE LEG STAND

During the explanation and demonstration, have the subject stand in the **"Rhomberg Position."** (Stand upright with heels and toes together, and hands at the side.)

TEST: From the **"Rhomberg Position,"** instruct the subject to first balance on his left leg by raising his right leg until his right foot is six inches off the ground. Have the subject point his toes down on the right foot, and while looking at his right foot, count in 1/1000s for 30 seconds out loud. (Have the subject count one thousand one, one thousand two, one thousand three, etc.) If at any time the subject loses his balance, he is to regain balance and continue counting where he left off. Discontinue test if subject is in danger of injury.

NOTES:

1. Note if subject uses arms or any other object for balance.

2. Note any difficulties in balancing.

3. The subject must count correctly.

4. Make sure the subject performs the test as instructed.

DRUG TESTING

FINGER TO THE NOSE

During the explanation and demonstration, the subject should stand in the **"Rhomberg Position."** (Stand upright with heels and toes together, and hands at the side.) Have the subject make a fist with both hands and extend his index finger on each hand, then place his arms at his sides.

TEST:
From the above position, instruct the subject to tilt his head back and close his eyes. When instructed, the subject is to touch the tip of his index finger to the tip of his nose. After touching his nose, the subject will bring his hand down to the starting position without being told. The sequence of instruction is left, right, left, right, right, left.

NOTES:
1. Note any body movements, such as swaying, body tremors, muscle rigidity, etc.

2. Observe where the index finger touches the face.

3. Make sure the subject performs the test as instructed.

DRUG TESTING

BODY FLUIDS REQUIRED FOR TESTING

All Narcotics:
(Heroin, Opium, Demerol®, Codeine.)

Urine (20cc) Blood is preferred

All Sedatives/Hypnotics:
(Barbiturates, Valium®, Librium®, Methaqualone.)

Blood (10ml-2 vacutainer tubes)

P.C.P.: Blood

Marijuana: Blood

L.S.D.: No Test

Cocaine/Amphetamines: Blood

DET, DMT, STP, DOM: Urine

NOTE: If you are unsure, it is advisable to take blood as the subject may be under the influence of a combination of drugs.

DRUG TESTING

LENGTH OF TIME DRUGS CAN BE DETECTED IN URINE

Cocaine
Metabolite* — 2-3 days

Cannabis:
Single Use — 3 days
Moderate Use (4 times/week) — 5 days
Heavy Use (Daily) — 10 days
Chronic Heavy Use — 21-27 days

Opiates
(Including Heroin, Morphine, Codeine) — 48 hours

P.C.P.
(Phencyclidine) — Approx. 8 days

Amphetamines & Methamphetamines — 48 hours

Benzodiazepines
(Including Valium®, Librium®-Therapeutic Dose) — 3 days

Barbiturates
Short Acting (Including Secobarbital) — 24 hours
Intermediate Acting — 48-72 hours
Long Acting
(Including Phenobarbital) — 7 days or more

Propoxyphene
(Including Darvon®)
Unchanged — 6 hours
Metabolite* — 6-48 hours

*Metabolite is the process of metabolizing. The body identifies the substance, uses the substance and excretes the substance. During this process the chemical make-up of the substance can change according to the drug used at the time.

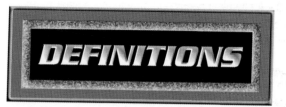

DEFINITIONS

ANALOG - A chemical compound structurally similar to another compound but differing often by a single element. The "new" compound may be several times stronger than the original compound.

BRUXISM - Grinding of the teeth.

CONJUNCTIVAE - Inner portion of the lower eyelid.

CONSTRICTION - When the pupil of the eye is small or smaller than normal.

CYCLIC BEHAVIOR - Mood swings, usually violent to passive and back to violent.

DILATION - When the pupil of the eye is large or larger than normal.

GAIT ATAXIA - Impaired stride while walking.

HALLUCINOGEN - A substance which produces hallucinations (apparent sensory experience of something that does not exist outside the mind).

H.G.N. - Horizontal Gaze Nystagmus.

HORIZONTAL GAZE NYSTAGMUS - The involuntary jerking of the eyes horizontally (side to side).

DEFINITIONS

NON-CONVERGENCE/STRABISMUS - The inability to cross eyes and hold on a fixed object.

NYSTAGMUS - An involuntary jerking of the eyeballs. Nystagmus occurs horizontally and/or vertically.

PARANOIA - Tendency on the part of the subject toward excessive or irrational suspiciousness and distrust of others.

PSYCHOSIS - Serious mental illness characterized by defective or lost contact with reality often with hallucinations or delusions.

PTOSIS - A drooping of the upper eyelid.

PUPIL - The round, black middle part of the eye. Regulates the amount of light that reaches the optic nerve.

PUPILOMETER - Gauge by which pupil size is measured in millimeters. (It is only a standard, not an exact measuring device)

REBOUND DILATION - A pulsation of thse pupils.

SCLERA - The white portion of the eye.

SYNESTHESIA - A mixing of senses.
    EXAMPLE: Hearing colors or seeing sounds.

STREET SLANG GLOSSARY

STREET SLANG GLOSSARY

STREET SLANG

Varies greatly from city to city, state to state, culture to culture, etc. We have attempted to gather the most commonly used language.

8-TRACK Street gang term meaning 2.5 grams of Cocaine

ABE Five dollars worth of a drug

ACAPULCO GOLD A particularly potent form of Marijuana grown in the Acapulco area (See GOLD and GOLD LEAF)

ACCESSORIES Drug paraphernalia

ACE 1) A Marijuana cigarette (See JOINT) 2) P.C.P.

ACID L.S.D. (Lysergic Acid Diethylamide)

ACID CUBE A sugar cube containing L.S.D.

ACID FREAK A heavy regular user of L.S.D.

ACID HEAD L.S.D. user

ACK-ACK Method by which Heroin/Cocaine is smoked on the tip of a burning cigarette

ACTION To use or sell drugs

AD A drug addict

ADAM Slang for the drug MDMA (3,4-Methylenedioxy-N-Methylamphetamine)

AFGHANI Drugs from Afghanistan Usually Marijuana

AMF Slang for the drug Alpha-Methylfentanyl

AMPED High on amphetamines

ANGEL DUST 1) Phencyclidine (P.C.P.) 2) P.C.P. sprinkled on Marijuana in powdered form and smoked

ANIMAL TRANK P.C.P.

STREET SLANG GLOSSARY

ARTILLERY Drug paraphernalia for injecting

ASTRO TURF Marijuana

AUTHOR A doctor or anyone who writes illegal prescriptions

BABYSITTER An individual knowledgeable about the effects of hallucinogens, particularly in the case of L.S.D. The babysitter provides reassurance and reality for the novice user (See CO-PILOT)

BACK-UP A procedure permitting blood back into the syringe to ensure that the needle is in a vein (a frequent precaution taken by veteran heroin addicts)

BAD TRIP An unpleasant, frightening or even terrifying experience occurring after the ingestion of a hallucinogenic drug or after ingestion of other drugs with hallucinogenic properties

BAG A small container of a drug, usually just enough for personal use

BALL Mexican Black Tar Heroin

BALLOON A toy balloon used for packaging Mexican Powdered Heroin. The balloon is used to enable the possessor to swallow it if approached by the authorities. It is later retrieved after defecation

BANG Injecting

BARBS Barbiturates

BARREL 1) A quantity of 100,000 pills 2) A particular shape of L.S.D. tablet

BASA Spanish word for base

BASE Freebased Cocaine

BASEBALL Cocaine Freebase

STREET SLANG GLOSSARY

BASINE The process of converting powdered Cocaine (Hydrochloride) into a purified solid for smoking

BASUCO/BASA Raw Coca Paste directly from the Coca Plant. It is a dark paste that is smoked, usually by South American peasants

BATU Hawaiian term for the large smokable crystals of Methamphetamine

BAYONET Hypodermic syringe

BEANS Dexedrine

BEAUTIFUL A drug of good quality, producing an exceptionally intense euphoria

BEHIND STUFF Using heroin, as in "I'm behind stuff"

BELLY HABIT Addiction where withdrawals cause severe stomach cramps

BELT 1) High or Euphoria produced by a drug high 2) To quickly consume alcohol 3) A large mouthful of alcohol.

BENNIES The prescription drug Benzedrine, however, it is no longer manufactured (See BENZ and DRIVERS)

BENT To be high on any drug

BENZ The prescription drug Benzedrine, however, it is no longer manufactured (See BENNIES and DRIVERS)

BERNICE Cocaine

BHANG Marijuana

BIG CHIEF Peyote

BIG C Cocaine

BIG D L.S.D.

BIG H Heroin

STREET SLANG GLOSSARY

BIG MAN Upper level drug dealer

BINDLE Paper used to hold a personal amount of a powdered drug Folded like an envelope

BINGE A sustained period of uninterrupted alcohol uses, sometimes refers to the same practice with other drugs

BLACK & WHITES Biphetamine that comes in a black & white capsule (See BLACK BEAUTIES)

BLACK BEAUTIES Biphetamine that comes in a black and white capsule (See BLACK & WHITES)

BLACK JACK Tincture of Opium cooked to a concentrated form and injected

BLACK TAR HEROIN A form of Mexican Heroin

BLANK An inert substance mixed with a drug to produce more of the substance for sales

BLASTED An intense drug high

BLOND Gold or yellow colored solid Hashish from the Middle East (Lebanese Blond)

BLOTTER ACID Small squares of heavy stock paper, perforated for tearing, with a drop of L.S.D. on each. Ingested orally. Sometimes there are pictures stamped on each one

BLOW 1) Slang for Cocaine 2) Inhalation of smoke

BLOW A STICK (OR JOINT) Smoking a marijuana joint

BLOW THE VEIN Injecting a vein with too much of the substance usually causing the vein to collapse

BLOW YOUR MIND To get high on a hallucinogenic

STREET SLANG GLOSSARY

BLUE CHEER A combination of L.S.D., Methamphetamine, and Strychnine

BLUE DEVILS Prescription drug Amytal Sodium in a blue capsule

BLUE HEAVEN L.S.D.

BLUES Amytal Sodium capsule

BLUE STAR A type of Morning Glory plant. The seeds can cause hallucinations similar to that of L.S.D.

BLUE VELVET Tincture of Opium added to powdered Tripelennamine, made into a solution and injected for a very intense high

BO Street gang term for Marijuana

BODY CARRIER Drug smuggler who carries the contraband in their clothes or on their body

BODY PACKER Drug smuggler who swallows the contraband which is usually wrapped in balloons or condoms. Later it is retreived after defecation

BOGART Not sharing any drug

BOMBED Excessive drug intoxication

BOLIVIAN 1) Cocaine of the purest form 2) Country of origin

BOLSA Spanish word for bag. Usually refers to Heroin

BOLT Amyl Nitrite

BONG Marijuana smoking pipe that is usually glass with a cooling chamber that is filled with water or wine

BOWL 1) Marijuana pipe 2) A degree measurement of Marijuana

BOTTLE 100 pills

BOY Heroin

STREET SLANG GLOSSARY

BRICK A quantity of Marijuana compressed into the shape of a brick that usually weighs a kilogram (2.2 lbs.)

BRING DOWN 1) To precipitate a "crash" from the excessive agitation produced by stimulants, via the ingestion of a CNS depressant 2) To help reduce highly adverse effects produced in some hallucinogen users via talk, reassurance, and sometimes minor tranquilzers

BRING IT UP To bulge a vein prior to injection

BRODY, TO THROW A To feign illness or withdraw in an attempt to obtain a narcotic prescription from a sympathetic physician

BROTHER Heroin

BROWN STUFF Mexican Brown Powdered Heroin

BROWNIES Regular fudge brownies mixed with Marijuana

BUD The blossom at the top of the Marijuana plant that contains the highest level of THC which is the active component of the plant

BUDDHA STICK Potent Asian Marijuana which is wrapped around bamboo sticks for shipping

BUFF/BUFFED 1) To dilute a drug 2) Muscular in appearance from use of steroids

BUG Itching sensation, due to cocaine overdose

BUGGER Black Tar Heroin

BULLET 1) Bullet-shaped plastic tube used for snorting drugs in the powdered form 2) One year jail term

BUMMED/BUMMER 1) Bad trip 2) A bad experience not necessarily drug related

STREET SLANG GLOSSARY

BUM TRIP A bad hallucinogenic drug experience

BUNK Low grade drug. Often the adulterant is solo and being represented as the drug

BURN Substances used to dilute potency of drug such as lidocaine, procaine, nicotinamide, or ephedrine

BURNED Cheated by a drug dealer

BURNED OUT In a state of brain or chronic behavior impairment resulting from chronic heavy drug use.

BUSH Marijuana

BUSINESSMAN'S LUNCH DMT, a hallucinogen with potent effects lasting 30-60 minutes

BUST An arrest by authorities and confiscation of drugs

BUTTON The top middle flower area of the Peyote Cactus (Hemispheric Taberculous). A hard, round object, slightly larger than a golf ball, containing the active ingredient of the plant, Mescaline, a hallucinogen

BUY A drug purchase

BUZZ A drug high

C Cocaine

C&H Cocaine and Heroin

CABALLO Spanish word for Heroin

CACTUS Peyote Cactus

CADET First time drug user

CALIFORNIA SUNSHINE L.S.D. produced and sold on the West Coast of California

STREET SLANG GLOSSARY

CAMEL Drug smuggler or drug carrier

CAN One ounce quantity of Marijuana

CANDY Cocaine

CANDY MAN Drug dealer or drug supplier

CAP Powdered drug in capsule form

CAP-UP To put powdered drugs into capsules

CARGA Spanish word for Heroin

CARRIER Drug smuggler or transporter

CARTWHEELS White Amphetamine tablets

CAT 1) Heroin 2) A synthetic designer drug, methcathinone, a stimulant with no medical application

CECIL/CEC Cocaine

CHANNEL Vein used for injecting drugs

CENT One dollar

CHAPAPOTE Spanish word for Mexican Tar Heroin

CHARAS Hindu for Marijuana

CHARGE The first effect of a drug high

CHARLIE Cocaine

CHASING THE DRAGON Heating Heroin or Opium on a piece of foil and inhaling the smoke

CHINA WHITE 1) Southeastern Asian Heroin 2) The synthetic opiate Alpha-Methylfentanyl

STREET SLANG GLOSSARY

CHIPPER/TO CHIP 1) An occasional drug user 2) To inject just under the skin

CHIPPING Taking narcotic analgesics on an occasional or irregular basis, not sufficiently often enough to become physically dependent

CHIVA Spanish word for Heroin

CHOPPING To dilute or adulterate a drug

CHRISTMAS TREES The prescription drug Tuinal

CIRCLES Rohypnol

CLEAN Drug free

CLUCK HEAD Street gang term for Cocaine addict

COASTING The euphoric high just after taking a drug, usually associated with Heroin

COAST TO COASTS Amphetamine tablets

COCAINE BLUES Depression from discontinuing use of cocaine

COKE Cocaine

COKE BUGS The sensation of bugs crawling under or on the user's skin associated with a Cocaine overdose

COKE HEAD A Cocaine user

COKE SPOON A small metal spoon used for snorting (inhaling) Cocaine

COKED OUT Excessive use of cocaine to point of incoherence

COKED UP Label for erratic behavior due to excessive use of cocaine

COLA Cocaine

COLD TURKEY Abrupt withdrawal from long term drug abuse

STREET SLANG GLOSSARY

COLUM Street gang term used for Colombian Marijuana

COME DOWN The gradual wearing-off of the effects of drugs

COME-ON The first feeling after taking a drug

COMMERCIAL Street gang term used for Marijuana

CONNECT/CONNECTION Drug dealer or supplier

CONTACT HIGH Mild euphoria occurring in non-smokers and believed by them to be the result of inhalation of the Marijuana fumes produced by smokers

COOK To prepare or heat a drug into liquid form in preparation for injection

COOKED High on drugs

COOKER 1) The container in which drugs are heated for injection. For example: Spoons, bottle caps, bottom half of a soft drink or beer can, etc. 2) One who manufactures drugs in a lab

COOKING COTTONS When a Heroin addict can not get Heroin, he will use the old cotton

COP To purchase drugs

CO-PILOT An individual knowledgeable about the effects of hallucinogens, particularly in the case of L.S.D. The Co-Pilot provides reassurance and reality for the novice user (See BABYSITTER)

CORINE Cocaine

COTTON A small amount of cotton used to filter impurities from dissolved Heroin as it is drawn into the hypodermic

COTTON, ASKING FOR Refers to an impoverished heroin addict to afford a "buy" scrounging the cotton used as a filter by other addicts that a very weak heroin solution can be made

STREET SLANG GLOSSARY

COTTON FEVER During the process of injecting, a small piece of cotton is used as a filter when the drug, usually Heroin, is drawn up into the syringe. Occasionally a fiber of cotton is drawn up into the syringe and is injected causing the user to become extremely ill

COURIER Drug smuggler or transporter

CRACK Cocaine Hypnochloride (powder) that has been processed into a pure solid form for smoking

CRACK HOUSE A structure where Crack (Freebased Cocaine) is sold

CRANK Methamphetamine

CRANKSTER User of Methamphetamine

CRANK BUGS The sensation of bugs crawling on or under the user's skin associated with a Methamphetamine overdose

CRAP 1) Heroin 2) Low quality drug

CRASH To abruptly stop using a drug

CRATE A large quantity of pills, usually 50,000

CRATER A deep flesh indentation at a particular site which has been subjected to repeated intravenous injections

CRINK Methamphetamine

CROKE To use Cocaine and Methamphetamine together

CROSS-TOPS Benzedrine tablets, so name for the crossed lines on one side of the pill as a result of the pill press mold.

CRYSTAL Methamphetamine

CUBE A sugar cube containing L.S.D.

CUT To adulterate or dilute drugs

STREET SLANG GLOSSARY

CYCLING Using different types of steroids one after another, but not at the same time. Example: Use a particular type of steroid for a period of time then use a different type of steroid to gain the maximum effect and reduce side effects

D L.S.D.

DAVA Heroin

DEAD PRESIDENTS Street gang term for money

DEAL/DEALER To sell drugs/One who sells drugs

DEXIES The prescription stimulant drug Dexedrine

DIAMONDS Amphetamine tablets

DILLIES Dilaudid (Hydromorphone)

DIME Ten dollars

DIME BAG Ten dollars worth of a drug

DIRTY 1) To possess drugs 2) To give a positive body fluid test

DIRTY PEE Positive urine test

DITCH WEED Low quality Marijuana

D.M.T. The synthetic hallucinogen Dimethyltryptamine

DO A LINE To snort (inhale) a "line" of a drug in powder form

DO UP To inject

D.O.A. Dead on arrival

DOLLAR One hundred dollars worth of a drug

DOLLY Dolophine (Methadone)

DOOBIE Marijuana cigarette (See JOINT)

STREET SLANG GLOSSARY

DOORS & FOURS Taking the prescription drugs Doriden and Tylenol w/Codeine #4 together. The effects are similar to that of Heroin

DOPE General term for drugs

DOPE FIEND Drug user

DOPER Drug user

DOSE 1) The amount of a drug taken 2) The amount of Methadone, a synthetic narcotic used to treat Heroin addiction, that is taken

DOSING Taking drugs

DOT A dose of L.S.D. so small it is hard to see

DOWNER Barbiturates or tranquilizers

DOWN, GET DOWN Inject a drug

DRAGGED A mild anxiety and fatigue state following Marijuana intoxication

DREAMERS Narcotic analgesic drugs

DRIVERS The prescription drug Benzedrine, however, it is no longer manufactured (See BENNIES and BENZ)

DROP To take a drug orally

DROP A TAB To take L.S.D. orally

DROP A DIME To inform on someone

DROPPER Hypodermic syringe

DRUGGIE Drug user

DRY 1) To be drug free 2) When the supply of drugs are low or gone

STREET SLANG GLOSSARY

DRY OUT To abstain from drugs or alcohol after a prolonged use, to the point of substantial or complete loss of tolerance

DRY UP When drugs, usually narcotics, are not available

DUCKETS Street gang term for money

DUST 1) A drug in powder form 2) Cocaine 3) P.C.P. (Phencyclidine)

DUSTED Under the influence of P.C.P.

DUSTER P.C.P. user

DUSTING Combining marijuana and heroin and rolling it in a form to be smoked

DYNO High quality drug

EAT To swallow drugs rather than be caught with them

ECHOES L.S.D. flashbacks

E/ECSTASY The synthetic drug M.D.M.A. (3,4-Methylenedioxy-N-Methylamphetamine)

EIGHT BALL 1/8 ounce of a drug

EIGHTH 1/8 of an ounce or a gram

ELEPHANT P.C.P. (Phencyclidine)

ELEVEN-FIVE-FIFTY Under the influence of a controlled substance California Health & Safety Code section violation **(11550 H&S)**

EMERALD TRIANGLE The California counties of Mendocino, Humbolt, and Trinity. This area is know for growing the high grade Sinsemilla Marijuana

EQUIPMENT Drug paraphernalia

EYE OPENER The first Heroin injection of the day

STREET SLANG GLOSSARY

FACTORY A location where illicit drugs are produced for street sale

FENTANYL A powerful anesthetic drug. Fentanyl may be diverted from hospitals for use. Analogs of fentanyl are usually manufactured illegally in clandestine drug labs

FINGER An amount of Marijuana or Hashish

FIRE A LINE To snort (inhale) an amount of a powdered drug

FIRE UP To light and smoke a Cocaine or Methamphetamine pipe

FIRED UP A drug high usually associated with Cocaine or Methamphetamine

FIT Paraphernalia for injecting drugs

FIVE CENTS Five dollars worth of a drug

FIX To inject a drug

FLAKE Cocaine

FLAKY Acting crazy

FLASH/FLASHING The first effect of a drug

FLASHBACK A reoccurrence of a drug usually associated with L.S.D. or P.C.P. The drug is stored in the fat cells and may reenter the body months or even years after the last ingestion

FLASH POWDER Methamphetamine

FLIP OUT To experience a severe psychological reaction to a drug

FLOATING Intoxicated

FLUFFING Chopping up Cocaine with a razor blade into a fine powder. It is then strained through mesh to increase its volume

STREET SLANG GLOSSARY

FLYING SAUCER Trade name for Morning Glory seeds

FOILING Placing a drug, usually Heroin, on a piece of tin foil, then heating it up and inhaling the smoke

FOURS 60 mg. Codeine tablets stamped with the number 4

FREAK One who chronically uses large amounts of a specific drug

FREEBASE Powdered Cocaine cooked and purified into solid form for smoking

FREEZE 1) Unavailability of drugs 2) Numbness caused by using cocaine

FRIED 1) Drug high 2) Close to an overdose

FRONT 1) To acquire drugs when payment is to be made by a reliable third party known to the seller 2) To purchase drugs on a short term credit

FRUIT SALAD A reckless combination of drugs

GANJA Hindu for Marijuana. Also used in the Jamaican culture

GAP To yawn (One of the earliest symptoms of heroin withdrawl)

GARBAGE Low grade drugs

GEE Gasket between needle and syringe

GEEZE To inject a drug

GET DOWN To use drugs, but is usually associated with Heroin

GET OFF The first effects of a drug

GHB Gamma hydroxybutyric acid (like liquid ecstasy). Illegal in U.S. except for medical research

GIRL Cocaine

GLASS Pure, solid, smokable form of Crystal Methamphetamine (See ICE)

STREET SLANG GLOSSARY

GOD'S MEDICINE Morphine

GO/GO FAST Outdated term for stimulant drugs, usually associated with Amphetamines

GOLD A particularly potent form of Marijuana grown in the Acapulco area (See ACAPULCO GOLD and GOLD LEAF)

GOLD DUST Cocaine

GOLDEN CRESCENT The Opium producing area of Southwest Asia (Iran, Pakistan, and Afghanistan)

GOLDEN TRIANGLE The Opium producing area of Southeast Asia (Burma, Laos, and Thailand)

GOLD LEAF A particularly potent form of Marijuana grown in the Acapulco area (See ACAPULCO GOLD and GOLD)

GOMA Spanish word for Mexican Tar Heroin

GOODS Refers to narcotics

GOOFBALLS Barbiturates

GRAM Common amount of a drug for personal use

GRASS Marijuana

GRAVEL Crack Cocaine

GRIFA Spanish word for Marijuana

GUIDE A baby sitter for an abuser of hallucinogenic drugs during an experience

GUN Injection paraphernalia

H Heroin

STREET SLANG GLOSSARY

HABIT Drug addiction

HALF 1/2 gram or 1/2 ounce of a drug

HAMMER COMING DOWN The rapid and dramatic transition from a normal feeling state to that which results from a full impact of a drug. Usually in reference to the effects of a drug intravenously administered

HARD DRUGS Narcotic analgesics. Also used to cover any drug which is controlled by a federal narcotic statutes, such as cannabis or cocaine

HANYAK Solid, smokable Methamphetamine

HAPPY DUST Cocaine

HARD STUFF Heroin

HASH The isolated active ingredient of the Marijuana plant

THC Hash comes in solid and oil form

HAY Marijuana

HEAD A heavy regular user of a drug. Reference is often made to a specific drug, such as "Acid Head"

HEAD SHOP A store that sells drug paraphernalia and other related drug items

HEARTS Dexedrine tablets

HEAVES Violent vomiting occurring during drug withdrawal

HEAVEN BLUE Trade name for Morning Glory seeds

HEMP Marijuana

HERB Marijuana

HIGH Drug induced euphoria

STREET SLANG GLOSSARY

HIT 1) Injection of drugs 2) A puff of a Marijuana Cigarette

HIT UP 1) To inject a drug 2) To borrow or attempt to borrow

HOG P.C.P. (Phencyclidine)

HOLDING To possess drugs

HONEY OIL Purified Hashish Oil containing the highest concentration of THC

HOOKA Marijuana smoking pipe or bong (See BONG)

HOOKED Addicted to drugs

HORN To snort (inhale) drugs in powder form

HORSE Heroin

HOT SHOT A very pure dose of Heroin which can result in death

HOUSEWIFE'S DISEASE Dependence on tranquilizers

HUBBA Cocaine Freebase

HUFFER A person who uses inhalants such as glue, paint thinner, petroleum products, etc

HUFFING The act of using inhalants

HUNTING Desperately seeking drugs prior to the onset of withdrawal

HUSTLING Addicts attempts to obtain enough money to purchase more drugs

HYPE Heroin addict

ICE Pure, solid, smokable form of Crystal Methamphetamine (See GLASS)

J Marijuana

JAB To inject

STREET SLANG GLOSSARY

JACKING OFF THE NEEDLE After putting the needle into the vein, some users pull the needle in and out of the wound to be sure the needle is still in the vein. This is usually associated with Heroin use

JAG State of being under influence of solvents

JANE Marijuana

JAR 1000 pills, also known as jug

JELLY Cocaine

JET FUEL P.C.P.

JIM JONES Street gang term for Marijuana cigarette laced with Cocaine and dipped in P.C.P.

JOINT Marijuana cigarette

JOLT The first effects of a drug

JONES A drug habit

JOY POP Irregular use of narcotics

JOY POPPING To inject just under the skin usually associated with Heroin use

JUG 1,000 pills

JUICE **1)** Cheap wine. More recently, liquid preparations of narcotic analgesic cough suppressants **2)** P.C.P. (Phencyclidine)

JUNK Diluted Heroin

JUNKIE Drug addict

JUNK WEED Low grade Marijuana

K Kilogram (2.2 pounds)

STREET SLANG GLOSSARY

KAKSONJAE Pure, solid, smokable form of Crystal Methamphetamine

KIBBLES & BITS Street gang term for small pieces of freebase cocaine

KEG 50,000 pills

KEESTER PLANT Drugs which are hidden in the rectum

KICK Stop using drugs

KILLER JOINT 1) Marijuana cigarette laced with P.C.P. **2)** Very potent Marijuana

KILLER WEED 1) Marijuana laced with P.C.P. **2)** Very potent Marijuana

KILO Kilogram (2.2 pounds)

KINGS HABIT The use of Cocaine

KIT Paraphernalia for injecting drugs

KJ P.C.P. saturated menthol cigarette (See KOOL JOINT)

KNOCKOUT DRUGS Liquid Chloral Hydrate and alcohol

KONA GOLD High grade Hawaiian Marijuana

KOOL JOINT Menthol cigarette laced with P.C.P. (See KJ)

KRYSTAL Crystal Methamphetamine

L L.S.D.

LACE To add a drug to another substance. Example: To spray P.C.P. on Marijuana for smoking

LADY Cocaine

L.A. TURNAROUNDS Amphetamines

L.B. 1 pound of a drug

STREET SLANG GLOSSARY

LEAF Marijuana

LEAPERS Amphetamines

LEB Lebanese Hashish

LIBS The prescription drug Librium

LID An ounce of marijuana

LIGHT UP To smoke marijuana

LINE An amount of a powdered drug laid in a thin line on a piece of glass or on a mirror approximately 2 inches long. This is usually associated with Cocaine use

LOADED Under the influence of a drug

LOADS Tylenol w/ Codeine #4 and Doriden

LOCO WEED Marijuana

LOVE DRUGS MDA, Methqualone

LOVELY P.C.P.

L.S.D. The synthetic hallucinogen D-Lysergic Acid Diethylamide

LUDES Quaaludes (No longer manufactured)

M 1) Marijuana 2) Morphine

M&M's M.D.M.A. (3,4-Methylenedioxyl-N-Methylamphetamine)

MAGIC MUSHROOM Refers to Psilocybin

MAKE A BUY Purchase drugs

MAINLINE To inject intravenously

MAN Drug dealer or drug connection

STREET SLANG GLOSSARY

MANICURE The removal of unusable parts of the Marijuana plant such as stocks, stems, seeds, etc

MANNITOL Cutter for cocaine

MARKS Puncture wounds or holes left from needle injection

MARKED UP Displaying puncture wounds from needle injections

MARY JANE Marijuana

MATCHBOX 1/ 2 ounce of marijuana

MAUI WOWIE High grade Marijuana from Hawaii

MDA Mellow Drug of America. The synthetic hallucinogen drug 3,4-Methylenedioxyamphetamine

M.D.M.A. 3,4-Methylenedioxy-N-Methylamphetamine is a synthetic hallucinogen with stimulant qualities

MEQUIN Methaqualone

MERCK Pharmaceutical Cocaine

MERSH Low grade Marijuana

MESC Mescaline

METH Methamphetamine

MEXICAN BROWN Mexican brown heroin

MEXICAN MUD Mexican Black Tar Heroin

MICKEY FINN The combination of the prescription drug Chloral Hydrate and Alcohol

MICRO DOTS L.S.D. on very small tablets

MIERA Spanish word for Heroin

STREET SLANG GLOSSARY

MIKE Microgram

MILK From milk sugar. Crystals of lactose frequently used in diluting Heroin

MIND-BLOWING Referring to a drug that produces extraordinarily powerful reaction. Usually a favorable experience

MINI BEANS Small Benzedrine tablets

MISS EMMA Morphine

MJ Marijuana

MMDA 3-Methoxy-4, 5 Methylenedioxyamphetamine which is a psychedelic Amphetamine

MONKEY The state of being in withdrawal from Heroin

MOTA Spanish word for Marijuana

MOUTH HABIT Oral drug use

MPPP One of the numerous, so called "Designer Drugs" similar to MPTP. Gives Heroin-like effects and can be made to look like White Heroin

MPTP Made from MPPP and is another "Designer Drug" with effects like White Heroin

MUD Mexican Black Tar Heroin

MULE A drug smuggler who actually carries the drugs

MUNCHIES Constant snacking associated with Marijuana intoxication

MUSCLING Injecting drugs into the muscle and is most commonly associated with steroids

NAIL Hypodermic needle

STREET SLANG GLOSSARY

NARC 1) A narcotics officer 2) An informer 3) To inform on someone, "To narc someone off"

NEBBIES The prescription drug Nembutal

NEEDLE FREAK One who injects drugs into the vein or skin

NEEDLE MAN An addict

NICKEL Five dollars

NICKEL BAG Five dollars worth of a drug

NINETEEN A term for speed. The nineteenth letter of the alphabet is "S"

NOD Being under the influence of Heroin. A relaxed state similar to sleep

NOSE CANDY Cocaine

NUKING THE COKE During the Cocaine Freebasing process the Cocaine Hydrochloride is mixed with baking soda and water, then heated. The microwave is used to speed up the process. A coffee maker machine may also be used

O 1) Cocaine 2) Opium

O.D. Overdose, usually a very serious condition

OIL 1) Hashish in oil form 2) Methamphetamine in oil form

OLLA Cocaine

ONE HITTER A drug that can only be diluted one time

ONE & ONE Two lines of Cocaine, one for each nostril

ON THE PIPE Street gang term for being addicted to Freebase Cocaine

OTC Over the counter. Refers to drugs that can be bought without a prescription

OUTFIT Paraphernalia for injecting drugs

STREET SLANG GLOSSARY

OUT OF SIGHT 1) Extraordinary quality, wonderful 2) A fantasic experience

OVERAMPED An overdose usually associated with a stimulant drug (Cocaine or Methamphetamine)

OZ/OZER One ounce

PAKALOLO Hawaiian for Marijuana

PANAMA GOLD High grade Panamanian Marijuana

PANAMA RED High grade Panamanian Marijuana that has a red color to the leaves and a red fuzz on the under portion of the leaves

PANIC 1) An acute state of fear precipitated by the onset of withdrawl and frantic action to acquire drugs 2) An abrupt drying up of heroin sources, affecting all local addicts

PAPERS 1) Marijuana rolling papers (Zig-Zag being the most common) 2) Blotter acid 3) A piece of paper folded like an envelope containing a small amount of a drug (See BINDLE)

PAPER ACID L.S.D.

PARTY BOWL/PARTY BONG A Marijuana pipe (See BONG)

PAREST Methaqualone

PASTA/PASTE Raw coca extracted from the coca leaves to be refined into Cocaine Hydrochloride. The raw coca is often smoked by the local peasants because of its availability and inexpensive price

P.C.P. Phencyclidine

P.D.R. Physician's Desk Reference. A book that contains all the pharmaceutical drugs. Used by doctors

P.C.E. N-Ethyl-1-Phenycyclhexylamine. An analog or member of the P.C.P. family of drugs

STREET SLANG GLOSSARY

PEACE WEED Marijuana laced with P.C.P.

PEAKING Reaching the highest point while under the influence of a drug

PEARL Cocaine

PEARLS Amyl Nitrite

PEANUT BUTTER CRANK Low grade crude Methamphetamine

PEDAZO Spanish word for Heroin

PEP PILL Amphetamine

PERCS The prescription drug Percodan

PERICO Spanish word for Cocaine

PERSIAN BROWN Raw, unprocessed Morphine sold on the streets as Heroin

PERSIAN WHITE High grade Persian Heroin

PERUVIAN FLAKE South American high grade Cocaine and refers to the shape of the Cocaine crystals

PEYOTL American Indian name for the Peyote Cactus

PHENNIES The prescription drug Phenobarbital

PIECE 1 ounce, or 1 pound, of a drug

PILL FREAK User of any type of pills

PILLOW 1) Methamphetamine 2) Package of 1,000 Amphetamine tablets 3) Methaqualone

PINNED Constricted pupils (the size of a pinhead) that result when under the influence of Heroin or other narcotics

PIN/PINNER A very thin Marijuana cigarette

STREET SLANG GLOSSARY

PINK HEARTS 1) Prescription drug Preludin 2) Fake stimulants that can be ordered out of magazines and contain Caffeine and/or Ephedrine

PINK LADIES The prescription drug Darvon

PINKS Seconal (named for the color of the capsule)

PLATEAUING Peaking out on a drug to the point where the user no longer feels the designated effects. Usually used to describe steroids

POLVO Spanish word for Cocaine

POP 1) To take a tablet orally 2) To inject subcutaneous

POPPERS Amyl and Butyl Nitrite, which is administered by crushing the small vile in which it is contained and immediately inhaling the vapors

POPPING 1) To swallow a drug 2) To inject a drug under the skin, not directly into the vein

POT Marijuana

POT HEAD Marijuana user

POWDERED Under the influence of Cocaine

P-2-P Phenyl-2-Propanone. A chemical used to make methamphetamine

PIPE-PEPERADINE A chemical used to make P.C.P.

PRIMO Street gang term for a Marijuana cigarette laced with Cocaine

PROCAINE Adulterant used to dilute the strength of cocaine or Mexican brown heroin. Has pharmacologica action of its own

PROP Phenly-2-Propanone. A chemical used for manufacturing Methamphetamine

PSYCHEDELIC A drug that distorts visual, auditory, and tactil senses

PUNTA ROJA High grade Columbium Marijuana

STREET SLANG GLOSSARY

PURPLE HEARTS Phenobarbital (Luminal tablets)

PUSHER Seller of drugs at the street level

Q'S Methaqualone

QUARTER 1) 1/4 gram of a drug 2) 1/4 ounce of a drug 3) $25.00 worth of a drug

QUARTER PIECE 1/4 ounce of a certain drug

RACK 2-5 capsules wrapped in tin foil

RAGWEED Low grade Marijuana

RAILS Lines of a powdered drug laid beside each other, on a mirror or a piece of glass, in preparation for snorting (inhaling)

RAINBOWS Tuinal (a combination of amobarbital and secobarbital) so called because of the bright red and blue capsules (see Red & Blues)

RAT An informer

RAVE PARTY Large party where attendees use hallucinogens. The drugs are often included with the price of admission

REDS/REDEVILS Seconal

RED & BLUES Tuinal. Bright red and blue capsules (see Rainbows)

REEFER A Marijuana cigarette

REGISTER To find the vein when injecting

RESIN The active ingredient of the Marijuana plant. THC (Delta-9-Tetrahydrocannabinol)

RIB Rohypnol

RIG The paraphernalia used to inject drugs

STREET SLANG GLOSSARY

RIPPED 1) Exhausted after a several day amphetamine run 2) Adversely affected by a drug

RIPPERS Amphetamines

RIPPED OFF 1) Robbed 2) Cheated in a drug buy

ROACH The butt end of a Marijuana cigarette

ROACH CLIP Any object used to hold the last bit of a burning Marijuana cigarette. An electrical alligator clip or surgical hemostat are commonly used

ROACHED OUT High on Rohypnol

ROCA Spanish word for Crack

ROCK Freebased Cocaine Hydrochloride

ROCK UP The process of converting Cocaine Hydrochloride to Cocaine base

ROCKET FUEL P.C.P.

ROIDS General term for steroids

ROID RAGE The uncontrollable, violent temperament displayed by some steroid users

ROLL 10 pills sold in tin foil

ROLLER PAPERS Cigarette rolling papers used to make Marijuana cigarettes

ROOFIES Rohypnol

ROOPIES Rohypnol

ROPE Marijuana

STREET SLANG GLOSSARY

RUBBY A skid row alcoholic who on occasion resorts to propyl (rubbing) alcohol

RUDERALIS Russian Marijuana plant. It has a low percentage of THC, the active ingredient in Marijuana

RUFFIES Rohypnol

RUMMY Skid row alcoholic

RUN A period of several consecutive days during which an individual uses Methamphetamines several times a day with little food or sleep

RUNNER Drug smuggler or transporter

RUSH An intense sensation which rapidly follows intravenous administration of such drugs as heroin, amphetamines or cocaine

SATIVA Marijuana. Comes from the scientific name Cannabis Sativa

SCHOOL BOY Codeine, so called because of the mildness of its effects when compared with the more potent narcotic analgesics

SCORE To make a successful drug purchase

SCRATCH Money

SCREENS Round metal mesh screens placed in a smoking pipe to hold the drug in the bowl

SCRIBE A person who writes false prescriptions

SCRIPT Drug prescription

SCRIPT WRITER Physician willing to write prescriptions for drugs

SECOS Seconal

SEND IT HOME To inject narcotic analgesics, cocaine or amphetamines intravenously

STREET SLANG GLOSSARY

SERVE Street gang term for selling drugs

SES Sinsemilla Marijuana (Sinsemilla means without seeds)

SET A combination of the prescription drugs Doriden and Tylenol w/Codeine #4

SET UP A situation in which undercover police officers entice a person to sell them drugs for the purpose of bringing about the person's arrest

SHABU Hawaiian word for the smokable form of Crystal Methamphetamine (See GLASS and ICE)

SHAKE The manicured leaves of a Marijuana plant

SHAVE 1) To adulterate, dilute or shortweight a drug 2) Literally shave off minute quantities and thereby shortweight the buyer

SHEET ACID L.S.D. on blotter paper (See BLOTTER ACID)

SHERMS A heavy-stock dark brown paper cigarette that is dipped into P.C.P. and then smoked (Short for Shermans)

SHIT Low quality drugs usually refers to Heroin

SHOOT-UP To inject intravenously

SHOOTING GALLERY A place where heroin addicts congregate to inject

SHORTCHANGED Having been sold drugs which are usually inferior in quality or purity

SHOTGUNNING Using any available steroid

SHOT IN THE ARM Although the general use of the term is now broader, it originally referred to an injection of narcotics, which is followed by a state of peacefulness, reverie and wellbeing

SHROOMS The hallucinogenic Psilocybin Mushrooms

STREET SLANG GLOSSARY

SICKNESS The onset of withdrawal

SKAG Heroin

SKIN POPPING Injecting subcutaneous

SKUNK WEED High grade Marijuana with a strong odor

SLAB A large, flat piece of Freebased cocaine

SLAMMING To inject. Usually refers to Heroin use

SLEEPERS Sedative/hypnotic drugs such as barbiturates

SLOW AND LOW Heroin users, when under the influence are said to be slow and low, in that they move slowly and speak in a low slow, slurred voice

SMACK Heroin

SMART DRINK Liquid concoctions containing various amino acids said to increase the intellegence of the user. Common at "rave" parties

SMASHED Heavily intoxicated with alcohol or other drugs

SMOKE Marijuana

SMOKE HOUSE A structure where users go to smoke Freebase Cocaine. They "rent" the pipes which contain the drug and leave the pipe behind

SNAPPERS Amyl or Butyl Nitrate

SNAPS Street gang term for money

SNIFF 1) To take cocaine, amphetamines or heroin by inhaling through the nose 2) To inhale solvents through both the nose and mouth

SNORT To inhale a drug in powdered form. Usually refers to Cocaine

SNOT Black Tar Heroin

STREET SLANG GLOSSARY

SNOW Cocaine

SNOW BIRD Cocaine

SNOW FLAKE Cocaine

SNOW BUGS The sensation of bugs crawling on or under the skin of a Cocaine user

SNOW SEAL A brand of non-porous smooth paper used to make bindles to carry drugs. Logo is a seal balancing a snowflake on its nose

SOAPER/SOAP Sopor (Methaqualone)

SOFT DRUGS Drugs of abuse other than narcotics also applied to those drugs perceived to have low toxicity and/or dependency liability

SOLES Slabs of solid Hashish

SOURCE A drug dealer or drug supplier

SPACE BASING Freebased Cocaine dipped in P.C.P. and then smoked

SPACED Unresponsive to the external environment, usually in reaction to altered consciousness produced by hallucinogenic drugs

SPACEY Referring to a strangeness or a state of psychic deterioration produced by excessive and/or heavy, chronic use of drugs

SPEED Injectable methamphetamine

SPEEDBALL Heroin plus cocaine

SPEEDFREAK Heavy regular use of injectable methamphetamine

SPEED LAB Laboratory where Methamphetamines are manufactured

SPEEDER Methamphetamine user

SPIKE Hypodermic needle

STREET SLANG GLOSSARY

SPOON 1) Small metal spoon used to snort (inhale) drugs in powdered form **2)** Teaspoon used to heat drugs prior to injection **3)** Street measurement of a drug, usually an amount for personal use and usually refers to Heroin

SPORE The reproductive part of the mushroom

SPORTING Cocaine use

STACKING The use of two or more steroids. One right after another, but not at the same time

STAR DUST Cocaine

STASH 1) A place where drugs are hidden to escape detection in the event of a sudden search by authorities **2)** To hide drugs rapidly when confronted with a search

STASH CANS Common brand name items, such as beer cans, motor oil cans, in which the bottom or top screws off and the drugs are hidden inside

STEP-ON To dilute a drug

STICK A Marijuana cigarette

STINK WEED Low grade Marijuana

STONED Pleasurably intoxicated

STOOLIE An infomer

S.T.P. Serenity, Tranquility, Peace. The synthetic hallucinogen 2,5-Dimethoxy-4-Methlyamphetamine

STRAWBERRY Street gang term for a female who exchanges sex for drugs

STRUNG OUT 1) In an emaciated and generally poor state of health and appearance due to chronic drug use **2)** Heavily dependent on drugs **3)** Sometimes to produce an extreme negative psychic effect during a single drug episode

STREET SLANG GLOSSARY

STUFF General term for drugs, specifically Heroin

SUGAR (MILK) HABIT Addict's desire for sweets due to heavy amount of milk mixed with everyday heroin

SUNSHINE L.S.D.

SUPER GRASS 1) P.C.P. laced Marijuana 2) High grade potent Marijuana

SUPER JOINT Marijuana cigarette dipped in P.C.P.

SUPER K The prescription drug Ketamine

SUPER WEED 1) High grade Marijuana 2) Marijuana laced with P.C.P.

SUPPLIER Drug dealer or drug source

SWEAT IT OUT To withdraw from narcotic analgesics

SWEEPING Snorting (inhaling) drugs in powdered form

SWING MAN A drug supplier

T The prescription drug Talwin

T'S AND BLUES Pentazocine (Talwin) plus tripelennamine prepared in a solution and injected

TABS L.S.D.

TAKE-OFF The first effects of a drug

TAR Mexican Black Tar Heroin

TASTE Sampling a drug before buying it

TATTOOING Prior to injecting, some users burn the end of the needle for sterilization. If the carbon deposits that form are not cleaned off prior to injecting, they will form under the skin causing dark marks. Same principle as a standard tattoo

TEA Marijuana

TEMPLE BALLS Hashish mixed with Opium then shaped into a small, round ball. Common in Nepal and parts of India

STREET SLANG GLOSSARY

TEN CENTS Ten dollars

TEN CENT BAG Ten dollars worth of a drug

THAI STICK Potent Marijuana from Thailand whose buds are attached to six inch sticks with string

THC Delta 9-Tetrahydrocannabinol. The active ingredient of the Marijuana plant

THRUSTERS Amphetamines

TIE A tourniquet tied around the arm to inhibit blood flow so the vein will bulge for injecting. Example: Belt, scarf, hose, surgical tubing, etc

TIE UP To apply a belt or tourniquet to the arm or leg to produce distention of a vein for an injection

TIE RAG (See TIE)

T.M.A. Trimethoxyamphetamine. Similar to M.D.A.

TOKE 1) A puff of a marijuana cigarette 2) To take a puff

TOKER Marijuana smoker

TOOLS Drug paraphernalia

TOOT Cocaine

TOOTER A piece of a drinking straw, a rolled up dollar bill, or other device used for snorting (inhaling) powdered drugs

TOPS The top buds of the Marijuana plant rich in THC

TOTALED Exhausted after an acute drug experience

TRACKS, TRACK MARKS 1) Collapsed veins resulting from chronic injection 2) discoloration and scars, resembling a tattoo in appearance, resulting from chronic injection

STREET SLANG GLOSSARY

TRANK P.C.P.

TRAVELER A user of hallucinogenic drugs

TREATMENT A dose of Heroin, especially when feeling the effects of withdrawal

TRIP Under the influence of a drug. Usually refers to L.S.D.

TRIPPERS L.S.D.

TUIES The prescription drug Tuinal

TURN ON 1) To produce a state of pleasurable excitement (the stimulas may be either a drug or other experience) **2)** To introduce someone to a drug or drugs

TWEAKED Under the influence of Methamphetamine sometimes refers to an adverse reaction

UNCUT A drug that has not been diluted

UP FRONT 1) As a sample, a small quantity of a drug is provided to the buyer to indicate quality **2)** As proof, showing the seller the money before the drugs are produced

UPPERS A general term used for most stimulant drugs of abuse, such as amphetamines, and related drugs. However, the term is not used for cocaine

UP TIGHT Tense, nervous or frightened because of a subjective experience produced by either a drug or by real events

USER Someone who uses drugs or is an addict

U.S.P. Pharmaceutical Methamphetamine

VALS The prescription drug Valium

STREET SLANG GLOSSARY

VAPORS Gang term for Freebase Cocaine smoke

VEGETABLE One who suffers from severe brain or behavioral impairment to the point of being unable to care for oneself

WACK 1) To dilute or cut a drug **2)** P.C.P.

WAKE-UPS Amphetamines

WASHBACK A method used to get any usable drug out of a pipe after it has been used several times (See WASHBACK METHODS, Page 161)

WASTED Exhausted after an acute drug experience, usually in reference to amphetamines or cocaine

WATER Methamphetamine

WATER PIPE A smoking pipe that has a chamber that is filled with water or wine. The chamber is used to cool the smoke (See BONG)

WEDGES Flat L.S.D. tablets

WEED 1) Marijuana **2)** Tobacco

WEEKENDER An occasional drug user

WET DADDIES P.C.P.

WHITE 1) Cocaine **2)** Asian Heroin

WHITE GIRL Cocaine

WHITES Amphetamine tablets

WHITE STUFF Heroin, usually Chinese

WINDOW PANE L.S.D. that is placed on small squares of gelatin

WIPED OUT To have lost consciousness from abusing drugs

STREET SLANG GLOSSARY

WIRED 1) Chronically dependent on amphetamines 2) Physically dependent on heroin

WIRED-OUT High on Cocaine or Methamphetamine

WITHDRAW The effects of quitting the heavy use of narcotics

WORKS Paraphernalia for injecting drugs

WRECKED 1) Exhausted after an acute drug experience 2) Having a very bad drug experience

X M.D.M.A.-(3,4-Methylenedioxly-N-Mtheylamphetamine)

XTC Also known as Ecstacy, MDMA, and Adam. Psychedelic drug common to "rave" parties

YELLOWS, YELLOW JACKETS Nembutal (Pentobarbital sodium)

YEN Agitated sleep occurring during withdrawal from heroin

Z One ounce of a drug

ZIP/ZIPPY Amphetamines

ZONKED Extremely high on drugs

DRUG ABUSE IN THE WORKPLACE

WORKPLACE DRUG ABUSE

DRUG ABUSE IN THE WORKPLACE

Statistics:

1. An estimated 70% of all individuals abusing drugs are employed.

2. The abuse of alcohol and other drugs is costing American business owners over one hundred billion ($100,000,000, 000) dollars annually due to insurance rate increases, workman's compensation, etc.

3. Drug use shows up at all levels in the workplace, from professionals to unskilled workers.

4. An estimated 20% of the workplace population is using alcohol or other drugs at the worksite.

5. Almost 60% of the worlds production of illegal drugs are consumed in the United States while only 5% of the world's population is located in the United States.

ABUSERS IN THE WORKPLACE ARE:

1. Less productive.

2. Miss several days of work.

3. More likely to injure themselves or someone else.

4. File more worker's compensation claims.

5. More likely to steal from employer and/or co-workers.

WORKPLACE DRUG ABUSE

ABUSERS IN THE WORKPLACE ARE (con't):

6. A cause of low morale among co-workers.
7. Cause an increase in co-worker's work load.
8. Cause insurance rates to increase.

RECOGNIZING ABUSERS IN THE WORKPLACE:

1. Accidents on the job.
2. Frequent absences and/or late to work.
3. Frequent mistakes that require additional work to correct.
4. Uncharacteristic behavior (moodiness, giddiness, violent threats, etc.).
5. Obsessed with drugs and alcohol and trying to get others to participate.

FIGHTING DRUG ABUSE IN THE WORKPLACE:

The best way to fight drug abuse in the workplace is through a five part program.

1. A written substance abuse policy.
2. An employee education & awareness program.
3. Supervisor training program.
4. An employee assistance program.
5. Drug testing when appropriate.

WORKPLACE DRUG ABUSE

RESOURCES FOR WORKPLACE DRUG ABUSE

California Narcotic Officers' Association
1(877) 775-6272
www.cnoa.org

American Council for Drug Education
1(800) 488-DRUG (3784)
1(301) 394-0600

Drug-Free Workplace Helpline
1(800) 843-4971 9 a.m. to 8 p.m. EST
1(800) WORKPLACE
www.health.org/workpl.htm

National Clearinghouse for Alcohol & Drug Information
1(800) 729-6686

National Institute on Drug Abuse Treatment (NIDA) Hotline
1(800) 662-HELP (4357)

The Resource Center for Alcohol & Drug Programs
1(800) 879-2772

APPENDIX

EARLY WARNING SIGNS

EARLY WARNING SIGNS OF ADOLESCENT DRUG ABUSE

There are numerous early warning signs of adolescent drug abuse. In order to detect the early warning signs, keep an open line of communication and be aware, observant, and open-minded. Drug abuse infiltrates all social, economic, and cultural structures. The current national average of the onset of drug and alcohol use is 12.8 years old.

EARLY WARNING SIGNS:

1. A distinctive change in attitude, usually a negative change.
2. Decline in school work and grades.
3. Poor school attendance, frequent Monday and Friday absences.
4. Distinctive change in friends.
5. Distinctive change in clothing.
6. Distinctive change in taste of music and movies.
7. Disciplinary problems at home and school.
8. Isolation from friends.
9. Mood swings.
10. Outbursts of violence (physical and/or verbal).
11. Discovery of drugs, drug paraphernalia, or drug publications.
12. Distinctive change in appearance. (Examples: tattoos, ear rings, nose rings, etc.)
13. Noticeable decrease in motivation and enthusiasm.
14. Abandonment of areas of interest or hobbies.
15. Stealing (inside and outside the home.)
16. Marked increase of physical illness.

GATEWAY DRUGS

Gateway drugs are most commonly used by adolescents. These drugs are:
1. Alcohol - All products.
2. Tobacco - All products (including smokeless).
3. Inhalants - All products.

Adolescence is the life-stage between childhood and adulthood. The onset of Gateway Drug use can begin as early as 12, but can vary. Adolescents use the so-called Gateway Drugs due to the fact they are so readily available and inexpensive. These chemicals can cause inhibition of growth and abnormal emotional development. The reason they are called Gateway Drugs is they can lead the adolescent down the path toward serious illicit drug abuse.

DRUG STATISTICS

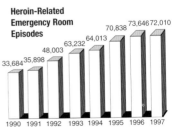

Heroin-Related Emergency Room Episodes

1990: 33,684
1991: 35,898
1992: 48,003
1993: 63,232
1994: 64,013
1995: 70,838
1996: 73,646
1997: 72,010

Source: Drug Abuse Warning Network 1999

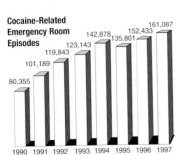

Cocaine-Related Emergency Room Episodes

1990: 80,355
1991: 101,189
1992: 119,843
1993: 123,143
1994: 142,878
1995: 135,801
1996: 152,433
1997: 161,087

Source: Drug Abuse Warning Network 1999

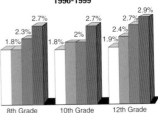

High School Students Who Ever Used Steroids 1996-1999

8th Grade: 1.8%, 2.3%, 2.7%, 1.8%
10th Grade: 2%, 2.7%, 2.7%, 2.9%
12th Grade: 1.9%, 2.4%, 2.7%, 2.9%

Source: Monitoring the Future Study 1999

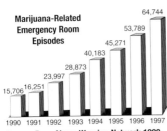

Marijuana-Related Emergency Room Episodes

1990: 15,706
1991: 16,251
1992: 23,997
1993: 28,873
1994: 40,183
1995: 45,271
1996: 53,789
1997: 64,744

Source: Drug Abuse Warning Network 1999

DRUG STATISTICS

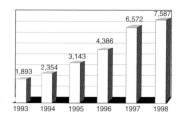

DEA Methamphetamine Arrests

1993: 1,893
1994: 2,354
1995: 3,143
1996: 4,386
1997: 6,572
1998: 7,587

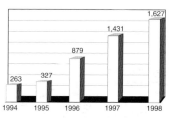

DEA Methamphetamine Lab Seizures

1994: 263
1995: 327
1996: 879
1997: 1,431
1998: 1,627

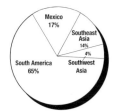

Mexico 17%
Southeast Asia 14%
Southwest Asia 4%
South America 65%

Heroin Signature Program
Source of Heroin Seized in the U.S.

The DEA's Heroin Signature Program (HSP) uses scientific profiling to identify the origin of heroin seized and purchased within the United States. Heroin from each of the world's four major source areas has a unique production process, or "signature," which DEA chemists use to determine if the drug is from South America, Mexico, Southeast Asia or Southwest Asia. In addition to source area identification, the HSP provides intelligence on wholesale purity and tracks transitions in heroin smuggling patterns into and throughout the nation. HSP data is used in conjunction with investigative intelligence and with drug production and seizure data to develop an overall assessment of the trafficking of heroin to and within the United States and alerts the agency to new drug threats. In 1991-1992, for example, drug couriers arriving at East Coast airports were bringing a new type of high-purity heroin that was different from all heroin previously analyzed. Many of the couriers were from Columbia, and DEA intelligence confirmed that opium poppies were being grown in Columbia. Comparative analysis of these samples are now compared. Associating source country authentic samples and intelligence reporting with the results of chemical analysis continually validates the program.

AIRCRAFT DRUG SMUGGLING

INDICATORS OF AIRCRAFT NARCOTIC SMUGGLING

Over the past few years, Puerto Rico, Florida, Louisiana, Texas, Arizona, New Mexico, and California have been flooded with persons and/or organizations attempting to smuggle large amounts of narcotics into the United States by air. The following indicators will help make you aware that smuggling of narcotics may be present, but not absolutely the case.

(1) Aircraft with passenger seats missing.

(2) Observing someone buying a large amount of aviation gas without an aircraft, or gas cans inside aircraft.

(3) Numerous cardbcard boxes, duffle bags, plastic bags, etc., inside the aircraft; seeds, green vegetable matter, fragments of various colored butcher or celiophane paper indicating possible marijuana debris visible inside the aircraft; tape markings or residue around aircraft tail number.

(4) Maps or other evidence of flights to Mexico, the Caribbean, Central or South America present in the aircraft when the pilot avoids reference to such flights, or a pilot requesting maps or information pertaining to areas in Mexico, the Caribbean, Central or South America when it appears he is not going to follow official procedures for such trips.

(5) Strong odors from the aircraft (perfumes and deodorizers are often used to disguise the odor of marijuana or cocaine).

(6) FAA registration numbers on the aircraft which appear to be incomplete, crooked altered, or concealed.

(7) Muddy wheels, dirty or dusty aircraft, beat-up props, pitted undercarriage, chipped paint on leading edges of wings and tail, or other evidence of landings and takeoffs on unpaved strips, fields, sand, etc.,

(8) Vans, panel trucks, or campers meeting the aircraft at an isolated location on the field.

AIRCRAFT DRUG SMUGGLING

(9) Pilot or passengers reluctant to leave the immediate area of the aircraft or to allow others close to the aircraft during refueling or servicing.

(10) Payment of cash for fuel or services, or display of large amounts of cash by the pilot or passengers.

(11) Persons who list themselves on aircraft rental applications as being self-employed and operating from their residence.

(12) Persons who rent hangars for one month or similar short-term basis, particularly when they pay cash in advance and give minimal information.

(13) Pilots who own or operate expensive aircraft with no visible means of support.

(14) Pilots reluctant to discuss destination, point of origin, or any of the above conditions.

Any of the indicators mentioned, especially when coupled with other suspicious behaviors by the aircraft operator or occupants, may indicate that the aircraft is being used for illegal activity.

Any of the indicators mentioned, especially when coupled with other suspicious behaviors by the aircraft operator or occupants, may indicate that the aircraft is being used for illegal activity.

When the indicators are observed and you feel there is a possibility that individuals might be engaged in smuggling, note any information regarding the identity of the pilot(s), other occupants, aircraft, description, and license numbers of vehicles. Under no circumstances should you take any direct action on your own. Immediately, or as soon as can be done safely, notify U.S. Customs. Use the national 1-800-BE-ALERT number or contact the nearest Customs Office of Enforcement. All information is held in confidences.

DRUG PREVENTION

RESOURCES FOR DRUG PREVENTION

DRUG PREVENTION ORGANIZATIONS

For the Office of National Drug Control Policy that includes drug prevention organizations for each state such as News & Public Affairs; Drug Facts & Statistics; Publications; National Drug Control Policy; Prevention & Education; Treatment; Science, Medicine & Technology; Enforcement; etc., visit:

California Narcotic Officers' Association
www.cnoa.org 1(877) 775-6272

NARCOTIC EDUCATION FOUNDATION OF AMERICA

The California Narcotic Officers' Association offers a series of very informative drug and narcotic information bulletins for the Narcotic Education Foundation of America (NEFA Bulletins). Each bulletin is 3 pages in length and make great educational tools. These bulletins are offered at no charge. Their duplication and distribution is encouraged by the CNOA. For downloadable versions of these bulletins, visit their above listed web site.

www.whitehousedrugpolicy.gov

OTHER DRUG ABUSE RESOURCES ON THE INTERNET

www.adhl.org

www.health.org

www.usdoj.gov/dea

www.drugabuse.gov

www.streetdrugs.org

http://members.aol.com/glskid/drugprevention.html

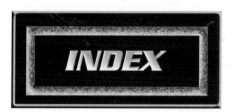

INDEX

A

Adapin, 35
Depressant Combinations. See also Combinations
Additional Inhalants, 66
Additional Narcotics, 102
Additional Stimulants, 130
Aerosol, 57, 61, 65, 66
Alcohol, 39, 42, 174, 175, 228, 229, 230, 232, 233
Alprazolam, 34
Amitriptyline Hydrochloride, 35, 37
Amobarbital, 32
Amosecobarbital, 32
Amphetamine, 2, 113, 115
Amytal, 32
Analog, 182
Anti-Anxiety Tranquilizers, 34
Anti-Depressants, 35
Anti-Psychotic Tranquilizers, 36
Atarax, 34
Ativan, 34

B

Barbiturates, 42, 179, 180
Biphetamines, 2, 115
Black Tar, 77
Brush Cleaner, 66
Bruxism, 113, 115, 117, 121, 125, 127, 129, 130, 182
Buticaps, 32
Butisol, 32
Butyl Nitrite, 2, 55

INDEX

C

Cannabis, 180
Centrax, 34
China White, 75
Chloral Hydrate, 33
Chlordiazepoxide, 34
Chlordiazepoxide & Amitriptyline, 37
Chlordiazepoxide Hydrochloride & Clidinium Bromide, 37
Chloroform, 66
Chlorohydrocarbons, 2, 57
Chlorpromazine, 36
Cibalith, 36
Clorazepate, 34
CO2 Cartridges, 66
Cocaine (Freebase), 3, 117
Cocaine (Powder), 3, 121
Cocaine Crack/Freebase Paraphernalia, 119
Cocaine Powder-Paraphernalia, 123
Cocaine Sifter, 134
Codeine, 3, 4, 68, 69, 179, 180
Combinations, 37
Come, 55
Computer Keyboard Dusters, 66
Conjunctivae, Definition of, 182
Constriction, Definition of, 182
Cooking Spray, 66
Copper Scouring Pads, 135
Correction Fluid, 4, 59
Crack (Cocaine), 117
Crack (Paraphernalia), 119
Crank, 127
Cyclic Behavior, Definition of, 182
Cylert, 130

INDEX

D

D.M.T., 5, 44, 45
Dalmane, 34
Darvocet, 102
Darvon, 102, 180
Darvon-N, 102
Demerol, 4, 70, 71, 179
Desipramine, 35
Desyrel, 35
Diazepam, 34
Didrex, 130
Dilation, Definition of, 182
Dilaudid, 5, 73
Dimethyltryptamine, 5, 44
Dolophine Sulfate (Methadone), 91
Doriden, 33
Doxepin Hydrochloride, 35
Droperidol, 36
Drug Lab, 136
Drug Prevention, 238
Dry Wash Method, 161

E

Ecstasy (XTC), 5, 109
Elavil, 35
Empty Aerosol Cans, 66
Equanil, 33
Eskalith, 36
Ethchlorvynol, 33

INDEX

Ether, 66
Ethinamate, 33

F

Fentanyl, 102
Fluphenazine Hydrochloride, 36
Flurazepam, 34
Freebase, 117, 135, 138, 161
Freebase (Cocaine), 3
Freebase Smoking Pipe, 137, 138

G

Gait Ataxia, Definition of, 182
GHB/GHL/GBL, 6, 38, 39
Glutethimide, 33

H

H.G.N., Definition of, 182
Haldol, 36
Haloperidol, 36
Hashish (Domestic), 6, 16, 17
Hashish (Middle Eastern), 6, 18, 19
HASHISH OIL (MIDDLE EASTERN), 7, 23
Hashoil (Domestic), 7, 21
Heroin, 81, 89, 139, 179, 180
Heroin (Asian-China White), 7, 75
Heroin (Black Tar), 7, 77
Heroin (Mexican Brown), 83
Heroin Columbian, 8, 79

INDEX

Heroin Paraphernalia, 81, 85
Horizontal Nystagmus Test, 171, 172
Horizontal Nystagmus, Definition of, 182
Hycodan, 102
Hydrocarbons, 61
Hydroxyzine, 34

I
ICE, 161
ICE (METHAMPHETAMINE), 10, 125
ICE Smoking Pipe, 142, 143, 144, 145, 146, 147
Imipramine, 35
Inapsine, 36
Ionamin, 130
Isocarboxazid, 35

L
L.S.D., 8, 49
Laughing Gas (Nitrous Oxide), 63
Librax, 37
Librium, 34, 179, 180
Limbitrol, 37
Lithium Carbonate, 36
Lithium Citrate, 36
Locker Room (Amyl/Butyl Nitrite), 55
Lomotil, 102
Lorazepam, 34
Lotusate, 32
Lysergic Acid Diethylamide, 8, 49

INDEX

M

Magic Mushrooms (Psilocybin), 13, 53
Marijuana, 9, 17, 19, 21, 23, 25, 31, 179
Marijuana Cigarette, 9, 27
Marijuana Plant, 9, 29
Marijuana Roach Clips, 141
Marplan, 35
Mebaral, 32
Mellaril, 36
Meperdine, 9, 87
Mephobarbital, 32
Meprobamate, 33
Methadone, 10, 89
Methadone Dolophine Sulfate, 90, 91
Methadone Identification Card, 92, 93
Methamphetamine (Crank), 10, 127
Methamphctaminc (ICE), 10, 125
Methamphetamine (ICE) Assorted Smoking Pipes, 147
Methamphetamine (ICE) Smoking Pipe, 142, 143, 144, 145, 146, 161
Methamphetamine Lab, 136
Methaqualone, 33, 42, 179
Methcathinone, 129
Methyprylon, 33
Mexican Brown, 85
Mexican Brown (Heroin), 83
Miltown, 33
Morphine, 11, 95, 180

INDEX

N
Nardil, 35
Nembutal, 32
Nitrous Oxide, 11, 63, 65
Noctec, 33
Non Convergence, Definition of, 183
Non-Barbiturates, 33
Non-Convergence Test, 172, 173
Norpramine, 35
Nortriptyline, 35
Nystagmus, Definition of, 183

O
Opium, 12, 97, 179
Oxazepam, 34

P
P.C.P., 12, 104, 105, 180
P.C.P. Oil, 12, 106, 107
Pamelor, 35
Paraldehyde, 33
Paranoia, Definition of, 183
Parnate, 35
Pentobarbital, 32
Percocet, 12, 99
Percodan, 13, 101
Permitil, 36
Perphenazine, 36, 37
Perphenazine & Amitriptyline Hydrochloride, 37

INDEX

Petroleum Products, 66
Peyote, 13, 51
Phencyclidine, 12, 180
Phenelzine, 35
Phenobarbital, 32, 180
Phenytoin Sodium, 34
Ping Pong Ball Gas, 66
Placidyl, 33
Pocket Dealers, 148
Pocket Drug Weighing Scale, 148
Poppy, 12
Prazepam, 34
Preludin, 130
Promazine, 36
Proxlixin, 36
Psilocybin (Magic Mushroom), 13, 53
Psychosis, Definition of, 183
Ptosis, Definition of, 183
Pupilometer, definition of, 183

Q
Quaalude, 33, 42

R
Rebound Dilation, Definition of, 183
Reposans, 10, 34
Ritalin, 130
Roach Clips (Marijuana), 141
Rohypnol, 13, 40, 41
rush, 81

INDEX

Rush ªAmyl/Butyl Nitrite, 55

S
Scales pocket, 148
Scales, Common, 149
Sclera, Definition of, 183
Secobarbital, 32, 180
Seconal, 32
Serax, 34
Snorting Spoon, 150, 156
Snorting Tube, 151, 152
Snorting Vial, 153, 154, 155, 156
Sodium Butabarbital, 32
Sparine, 36
Speed, 10, 127, 175
Spray Paint (Silver), 66
Stash Cans, 157, 158, 159, 160
Strabismus/Non Convergence, Definition of, 183
Symptoms (Depressants), 42
Synesthesia, Definition of, 184

T
Talbutal, 32
Talwin, 102
Thai Stick, 14, 31
Thioridazine, 36
Thorazine, 36
Tofranil, 35
Tranquilizers, 42
Tranxene, 34

INDEX

Tranylcypromine, 35
Trazodone, 35
Triavil, 37
Trilafon, 36
tube, 123
Tuinal, 32
Tussionex, 102
Tylenol W/Codeine, 3, 4, 68

V
Valium, 34, 179, 180
Valmid, 33
Vazepam, 34
Vistaril, 34

W
Washback Method, 138, 161
Wet Wash Method, 161

X
Xanax, 34
XTC, 5, 109, 111